7 Keys to Lifelong Sexual Vitality

7 Keys to Lifelong Sexual Vitality

The Hippocrates Institute
Guide to Sex, Health, and Happiness

BRIAN R. CLEMENT, PhD, NMD, LN
ANNA MARIA CLEMENT, PhD, NMD, LN

FOREWORD BY GEORGE W. YU, MD

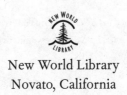

New World Library
Novato, California

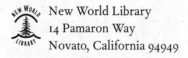

New World Library
14 Pamaron Way
Novato, California 94949

Text design by Tona Pearce Myers

Library of Congress Cataloging-in-Publication Data
Clement, Brian R., date.
7 keys to lifelong sexual vitality : the Hippocrates institute guide to sex, health, and happiness / Brian R. Clement, Anna Maria Clement.
    p.   cm.
Includes bibliographical references and index.
ISBN 978-1-60868-092-4 (pbk.)
1. Sex (Psychology)—Health aspects. 2. Sex. 3. Mind and body. 4. Nutrition.
I. Clement, Anna Maria. II. Title. III. Title: Seven keys to lifelong sexual vitality.
RA788.C44 2012
613.9—dc23   2012007127

First printing, June 2012
ISBN 978-1-60868-092-4
Printed in the USA on 100% postconsumer-waste recycled paper

New World Library is proud to be a Gold Certified Environmentally Responsible Publisher.
Publisher certification awarded by Green Press Initiative. www.greenpressinitiative.org

10 9 8 7 6 5 4 3 2 1

Contents

Foreword

One recent holiday season, I met with Drs. Brian and Anna Maria Clement on a project examining gene expression and the effect that the Hippocrates Health Institute lifestyle has on altering it. They graciously invited me to their holiday party, and I watched Anna Maria and Brian dancing to tune after tune as a young couple in love, totally oblivious to everything except the moment.

Knowing their heavy daily workload and the perpetual international and national speaking tours that they conduct, I was impressed by the apparent love they displayed despite their bigger calling and commitment to helping humanity.

Drs. Brian and Anna Maria have been the backbone of the renowned Hippocrates Health Institute through both thick and thin for years now. For the first time, they are further expanding to accommodate the global audience that attends their Florida-based program.

Over several decades of working with hundreds of thousands of people, they began to observe that more than food affects the health and longevity of individuals. Biological sexuality is intimately woven into the physical and mental health of all people. Together they began to accrue stories, science, and statistics on how central sex is in our lives. They also concluded, as they explain in this pinnacle book, that the moral codes of our civilization limit public discussion about sexuality. Yet, in all civilizations, the power of sexuality has always been present and acknowledged to a greater or lesser degree.

In my Asian culture, the *yang*, the male force, and the *yin*, the female force, should be balanced within every human being. The *chi* of sexual energy that binds us together is what perpetuates humanity. Sexual energy is the foremost driving force throughout life, even well beyond our reproductive years. But sexuality is more than the drive that triggers the physical act of intercourse. It is more the combined force of energy that is manifested by the unification of two committed, loving souls. Emotional, physical, and even spiritual well-being is the reward that one gains by expressing this foundational drive.

For more than three and a half decades, I have worked as a urological surgeon, with an intense focus on sex hormones, aging, health, and disease. Among my research projects was one that studied why centenarians such as the Okinawans of Japan have such remarkably high hormone levels compared to North Americans and Europeans. We found this to be true among the Okinawans' healthy population well into their seventies, eighties, nineties, and even their hundreds. As we observed the oldest generation of the longest-living humans on earth, it became clear that their low-calorie diets (1,500 to 1,800 calories per day) influence their well-being.[1] They consume a primarily plant-based cuisine from land and sea. They are mentally and physically active, playing sports and games, and they do not permit social boundaries between different age groups. Okinawans are radically distinct people, yet genetically close to the original Taiwanese. They are happy and healthy people, with well-defined facial features and small frames.

Merging the science of longevity with these observations, we can see that there is now growing, unshakable evidence showing that life extension, vitality, and sexuality are all enhanced via proper food and healthy minds. We can also predict that people living in this way not only desire and achieve more sexual intimacy, but do so much longer than the rest of us.

Given my background in biology, chemistry, medicine, and evolutionary biology, my viewpoint is that we humans are as primal as all other creatures, with the same core biological goals of survival and procreation.

Our sex hormones are tuned to these goals both before and after the reproductive years. Between the ages of twenty and forty, production of sex hormones, which also affect the adrenal and thyroid glands, begins to slow, and later it declines abruptly for women during menopause and, yes, for men during andropause.

In some ways, evolution has not caught up with our modernization. Modern conveniences such as electricity, heated homes, refrigeration, garments that keep us warm, and, above all, diagnostic medicine, which helps us identify disease before it kills, have helped to prolong the reproductive years. So what can we do about this evolutionary lag? Sex hormones are powerful body signals that can enhance or hinder our overall health, in addition to their controlling influence on sexuality and reproduction.

Drs. Clement begin the dialogue with the influence that food has on sex. They point out that positive nutritional factors such as minerals, vitamins, and proteins from plant fare, as well as whole food supplementation, help to sustain and increase sex hormone activity. They also explain that toxins in air and water, pesticides, fungicides, and herbicides — and generally the plethora of chemicals spewed around the globe — act to distort, weaken, and neuter healthy endocrine function and hormonal activity. This adds up to sexual dysfunction, which, when chronic, halts the biological and psychological desire to procreate.

What you will find quite interesting is the importance Drs. Clement place on the senses. Foreplay, including touch, fragrance, massage, erotic creativity, and emotional intimacy, starts the endocrinal engines and helps sex hormones to do their work. You can further enhance the act of love by preparing your body via pelvic exercise, yoga, visualization, tantra, and Taoism, as well as the totality of healthy living practices. It is refreshing to read the Clements' recommendations on how to enhance your sexuality without unhealthy practices.

There is no doubt that this book is one of the most important contributions to the betterment of sex. *7 Keys to Lifelong Sexual Vitality* is a clear and concise guidebook leading us back to sanity. When you read and embrace some of these commonsense suggestions, you will then possess the ability to differentiate distortion, cultural dogma, and outright craziness about sex from the sacred, biologically driven desire for intimacy in a committed relationship.

— George W. Yu, MD,
coauthor of *Critical Operative Maneuvers in Urologic Surgery*
and founder of the George W. Yu Foundation for Nutrition and Health

Healthy Sex Is Potent Medicine

Sex is like air;
it's not important unless you aren't getting any.

— Anonymous

Sexual energy is a universal fuel of life. It nourishes the human mind, body, and spirit. Besides diet and exercise, nothing will naturally enhance your health throughout your life more than remaining sexually active. Healthy sex is one of nature's most potent medicines.

This book takes a fresh scientific look at the physiological and psychological benefits of sexual intimacy, especially when it occurs in relationship with a committed partner. The information in this book will show you how to transform the sexual act from a mindless pleasure into a mindful health principle.

During our more than three decades directing the Hippocrates Health Institute, it has become increasingly clear to us that people who no longer have sexual intimacy in their lives tend to develop a range of health disorders, both physical and mental, more readily than those who remain sexually active. By contrast, our guests who have completed the Hippocrates program and continue its dietary regimen at home overwhelmingly report to us that their sex lives have improved beyond all measure.

We have also seen firsthand at Hippocrates that people in committed relationships who maintain sexual intimacy have three times the chance of achieving their health recovery goals than do people who are alone and not sexually active, or who are trapped in relationships without sexual intimacy. Our observations in this regard are supported by numerous medical studies — all detailed in this book — showing that individuals in long-term sexually intimate relationships live longer than most other people.

Sexual Dissatisfaction Is Global

When the Rolling Stones sing, "I can't get no satisfaction," does the lyric hit home with you?

If you're a married man, one out of three of you feels sexually frustrated.

If you're a married woman, one out of every four of you fails to experience the level of sexual satisfaction that you desire.

That's according to the Global Better Sex Survey, conducted among 12,563 people in 27 countries, including the United States. The results were presented to the European Association of Urology and published in the June 2007 issue of *Urology Times.*[1]

Half of those surveyed were forty years of age or younger. The most surprising finding of all was that one out of every two men confessed that they were unable to naturally maintain an erection long enough to satisfy their partner during intercourse.

Thoughts Have Biological Consequences

Sex is a natural experience that is essential to health. Your body has the biological urge for sexual release with or without your consent. If you don't give consent and cooperate, if you persistently repress your sexuality, or if you try to channel this sexual energy in a manner that isn't in alignment with your morals or your heart, the resulting conflict and friction between your mind and body will create health problems for you.

But if your mind affirms and supports your body's need for sexual expression, you will intensify your enjoyment of sex while multiplying its benefits to your health.

Books such as those by cell biologist Bruce Lipton (*The Biology of Belief*) and Georgetown University Medical Center professor Candace Pert (*Molecules of Emotion*) have persuasively made the case that our thoughts, beliefs, attitudes, and emotions directly influence the biochemical and cellular levels of our brains and the rest of our bodies.[2] It's a tightly woven feedback loop. The brain — and through it, our positive and negative thoughts and subconscious conditioning — controls the functioning of our cells, especially immune cells, which determine our state of health. This same process applies to our sexual health.

Men's and women's hormone secretions are one of the ways we communicate with each other at the level of the subconscious mind. The attempt to suppress this normal biological activity can create fear and abnormalities. Instead of being a delightful and normal experience, the sexual act is turned by repression into a kind of abomination that is whispered about or that becomes a source of embarrassment and scatological humor.

Prejudices about sex have created much of the social disharmony we see around us. A lot of the anger and violence exhibited in the world today can be traced to repressed or warped sexuality.

Sex Enhances Your Health

Sexual activity reduces depression and anger, anxiety and stress. It releases chemicals into the body that reinforce your immune system. It even improves your memory by producing chemicals that help to create new dendrites, which facilitate neuron communication in the brain.

Sexual intimacy is the key to attaining health and happiness. Ovarian cancer is related to infrequency of sexual release. So is prostate cancer. There is also a connection between sexual loneliness and a higher risk of early mortality. In this book, we also emphasize that sexuality must be handled with the greater good of humankind in mind. To carelessly impregnate a woman, for example, turns the sexual act into a cause for grief instead of celebration.

Once sex is demystified, once its extraordinary health benefits are known, it's our hope that people will become more inclined to drop their judgments about it. That is one of our key motivations for writing this book.

Diet Affects Your Sex Life

Sex is the most interesting of all subjects for human beings. We know of no topic that is more enchanting. Yet how open are we to discussing it honestly among friends and relatives, much less with strangers in public? Probably the second most popular subject to think or talk about is food. And in this book, you will learn how good food produces good sex.

There has always been a close relationship between food and sex. If healthy food is medicine — and it most certainly is — then healthy sex is potent medicine, too. Sex is as important a fuel to the human spirit and soul as good food is to the human body.

As nutritionists, we can tell you exactly which minerals, vitamins, proteins, and fatty acids the body requires to develop cells and structure. Many of these are sexual nourishment nutrients, too. They are essential to the production of the type of hormones and blood cells that allow us to have sexual intimacy. Without good blood flow to the genital areas, or adequate production of sex hormones, sexual vitality is beyond the reach of most people, especially our oldest citizens. We will explore the foods and herbs that naturally increase libido and enhance sexual performance, without the side effects associated with prescription drugs such as Viagra.

An inadequate diet combined with exposure to toxins can sabotage the greatest blessing of all bestowed by sexuality: the ability to conceive a child and bring new life into the world. Fertility difficulties are a huge and growing problem for couples. Anywhere from 12 percent to 33 percent of them, depending on which expert's estimate you accept, cannot conceive.

4

Toxins play a role in thwarting fertility, just as a nutrient-rich diet can help to regenerate it. We have had hundreds of cases of people who came to Hippocrates with fertility problems and subsequently overcame that challenge by using the healthy lifestyle that we teach.

During our decades of work with thousands of people facing health challenges, we have seen people who developed cancer primarily as a result of sexual frustration. As noted earlier, science is showing us that the risk of prostate cancer and ovarian cancer can be reduced if you have regular sex. But it goes beyond that. The psychology of sexual frustration and repression influences the physical biology of *all* illness and disease. We will show you how our immune systems suffer when our sex hormones aren't regularly stimulated.

For healthy sexual function, we must also have a physique that functions properly and at its optimal level. Our weight should be in a generally healthy but wide range: somewhere between obesity and emaciation. Bodily self-loathing of any sort tends to sabotage sexual desire and expression, and it undermines the very nutritional needs that keep our bodies from deteriorating.

Sex Can Lengthen Your Life Span

Intimacy gives people not only sexual virility but mental virility as well. The physical benefits of sex include higher levels of hormonal activity — allowing the body to grow healthier and stronger.

The hormonal symphony that arises from the sexual act, particularly in a committed relationship, instills an unsurpassed vitality. You'll never be closer to another human being, other than the time spent in your mother's womb, than when you are making love with that cherished partner.

As you and an intimate partner age together, the continued biochemical exchange of sexual union will fortify your health and extend your lives. The medical evidence presented in these pages overwhelmingly supports the life-extension powers of sexual vitality.

The Hippocrates Program Structure:
Your 7 Keys to Lifelong Sexual Vitality

At the Hippocrates Health Institute, our goal for more than a half century has been to educate our guests about how they can best empower themselves for their own self-healing. Our program is a holistic approach to health that combines these and other elements: detoxifying the body; providing the body with pure whole-food nutrients; offering massage, meditation, and exercise to further boost immune system activity; and, finally, using psychotherapy to remove mental roadblocks to wellness. This entire prescription — which in this book we identify as the "7 Keys" — works effectively whether your goal is to heal yourself from an illness or disease or to regenerate your sexual vitality for greater pleasure and a longer life. In this book, we have devoted one chapter to each of the keys, as follows:

Key One. Understand Your Sexuality: *What you may not have realized*
Key Two. Imagine Your Sexuality: *What you may not have visualized*
Key Three. Express Your Sexuality: *What you may not have*
acted upon
Key Four. Protect Your Sexuality: *What you need to guard against*
Key Five. Nourish Your Sexuality: *Which nutrients you need to absorb*
Key Six. Enhance Your Sexuality: *Which exercises you need to practice*
Key Seven. Prolong Your Sexuality: *Which lifelong health benefits*
you will gain

This book builds upon the Hippocrates Health Institute's program, showing you how mindful sexual activity can influence your overall health, your quality of life, and the length of your life. So that you can get the most benefit out of the medical science, nutritional data, and other advice in these pages, we ask only that you try to keep an open mind. Experiment and find what works best for you.

We're personally committed to the message in this book. While we're physician nutritionists and health educators rather than sexologists, our deep and longstanding insight into the dysfunction that people suffer in the realm of sexuality is what motivated us to write this book. Thousands of firsthand examples have shown us that when sexual health fails to flourish in a relationship or in a person's life, this failure becomes a significant contributor to premature aging and disease.

It's often said that happiness is a journey, not simply a destination. Being able to experience lifelong sexual vitality not only will enhance your prospects for happiness but will give your life's journey a renewed purpose and meaning.

Understand Your Sexuality

When authorities warn you of the sinfulness of sex,
here is an important lesson to be learned.
Do not have sex with the authorities.

— Cartoonist Matt Groening

A Quiz about Your Sexual Reality

One half of the world cannot understand
the pleasures of the other.

— Novelist Jane Austen (1775–1817)

The following series of paired statements challenges you to consider the ways in which you might sabotage your own sexual fulfillment, and maybe even thwart the sexual potential of the people in your life whom you most care about. Read each pair and circle the statement that more accurately reflects your feelings. Your responses may help to reveal the extent to which your beliefs, attitudes, and judgments about sexuality contribute to sexual dysfunction, absence of intimacy, or health problems related to sexual repression and frustration.

Sex is an energy I control.	or	*Sex feels like uncontrollable energy.*
Sex is always my choice.	or	*Sex often feels like an obligation.*
Sex feels nurturing.	or	*Sex feels hurtful.*
Sex feels like I am sharing with someone.	or	*Sex feels like I am "doing something to" someone.*
Sex requires communication.	or	*Sex needs no communication.*
Sex should be private.	or	*Sex should be secretive.*
Sex must be respectful.	or	*Sex can be exploitative.*
Sex should be mutual.	or	*Sex can be selfish.*
Sex should feel intimate.	or	*Sex can be emotionally distant.*
Sex should have boundaries.	or	*Sex doesn't have to respect boundaries.*
Sex empowers me.	or	*Sex means I have power over others.*
Sex reflects my values.	or	*Sex compromises my values.*
Sex enhances my self-esteem.	or	*Sex often feels shameful to me.*

The left-hand column lists healthy sexual attitudes. The right-hand column lists negative attitudes, which may be symptoms of sexual abuse or sexual addiction.

How Do You Define *Normal*?

Chastity — the most unnatural of all the sexual perversions.

— Philosopher Aldous Huxley (1894–1963)

Can you imagine having a sexual relationship with a robot? Will such liaisons ever be considered "normal"? These may seem like silly questions, but one day soon, probably within our lifetimes, sex with artificial partners will be a common topic of conversation. The technology to make such sex happen already exists.

If you saw the 1970s movies *Westworld* and *Futureworld*, in which humanlike robots provide entertainment and companionship for humans in settings that resemble Disneyland for adults, you know what we're talking about. The theme was developed even further in the 1980s in Ridley Scott's film *Blade Runner*, with a category of robots called replicants.

Will a robot be classified under future law as a mere piece of property, as a consenting adult, or as a sex slave? Will humans become psychologically and emotionally attached to them in ways we currently don't when using an inflatable sex doll or a vibrator?

Artificial intelligence researcher David Levy, at the University of Maastricht in the Netherlands, predicts that not only are love and sex with robots inevitable, but the first government to legalize human-robot marriages will be that of Massachusetts, via their Institute of Technology. The first groups of people inclined to take advantage of sex and marriage with robots will be thrill-seekers, people who are extremely introverted, those who have psychological problems, or those who feel too ugly to attract a desirable human mate.[1]

We must keep in mind that just a century ago interracial marriages were illegal in most of the United States, having been defined as "abnormal" and a "crime against nature." The same has been true with same-sex marriages, though that prohibition, too, is being abandoned as people's attitudes change about what is considered normal sexual behavior.

What we challenge you to do in this chapter is to begin thinking outside your comfort zone. What sort of nonviolent sexual relations between consenting adults do you find repugnant? What kind of nonviolent sexual acts do you refuse to engage in because of your upbringing? Unless we honestly examine our own inhibitions, we cannot discover the limitations on our full potential for expressing and experiencing a healthy sex life.

Sexual Practices around the World

Sexual practices defined as "normal" vary by country and culture. That much we know. But a study in a 2001 issue of the journal *Sexual and Relationship Therapy* makes this clear: "Except in a very few countries, we have no idea what people do in bed."[2]

Sexual desires are difficult to categorize based on "normal" versus "abnormal" standards. "Some people are attracted to mature or older partners, some to young adults," observes University of California, San Diego, biology professor Simon LeVay in his book *The Sexual Brain*. "Some go for skinny, some for fat. Some are turned on by candlelight and soft music, others by whips and abuse. Some are aroused by animals, some by motorbikes, some by corpses. Some like sex in groups; for others the ultimate sex object is their own body. There are even people who never experience sexual feelings of any kind."[3]

Little or nothing is known about what generates our sexual preferences, but here, culled from their studies, is some of what sex researchers do claim to know about worldwide sexual habits:

- In the United States, 30 percent of men and 28 percent of women say they are either celibate or have sex only a few times a year.
- In Britain, an average person has sex 2,580 times with five different partners during his or her lifetime.
- In India, many couples abstain from sexual activity after fifty years of age, particularly after a woman becomes a grandmother.
- Among sexually active sixteen- to forty-five-year-olds, the French have sex an average of 141 times a year, the highest rate among the countries measured, while residents of Hong Kong make whoopee only fifty-seven times annually, the lowest of any group.
- In many South American countries, teenage girls are taught by their mothers how to simultaneously remain "virgins" and satisfy sexual desires by engaging in heterosexual anal intercourse, rather than vaginal penetration, until they marry.
- An estimated 3 to 4 percent of the world's male population, and 2 percent of the female population, live exclusively as homosexuals. Within the animal kingdom, some percentage of the populations of about 450 species of mammals and birds engage in same-sex activities.

- Homosexuality remains illegal in fifty countries around the world, eight of which make homosexual acts punishable by death: Afghanistan, Iran, Pakistan, Mauritania, Saudi Arabia, Sudan, the United Arab Emirates, and Yemen.

- At least 60 percent of all couples in the world had their marriages arranged by their parents or other family members. The divorce rate among arranged marriages is a fraction of that among couples who marry for romantic reasons. The highest divorce rates are in Hungary and the United States, and the lowest in Afghanistan and India.

- Adultery among couples (at least instances that are confessed to in surveys) varies from 50 percent of Americans, 42 percent of the British, 40 percent of Germans, and 36 percent of the French (despite their reputation as philanderers) to 22 percent of Spaniards. Four countries exact the death penalty (on women, not men) for adultery — Iran, Pakistan, Saudi Arabia, and Yemen.[4]

Infamous Sex Myth

Premarital Sex Is More Common Today Than It Was in the Past

It may come as a surprise, but your parents and grandparents were just as likely to have had sex before marriage as you and your own children are. That's one of the findings from a 2007 sex study in the journal *Public Health Reports*.

"The likelihood that Americans will have sex before marriage has remained virtually unchanged since the 1950s," concludes the report.

Among women born in the 1940s, about nine in ten had sex before marriage. Today that figure remains the same, although there is one big difference: out-of-wedlock births are much higher now than a half century ago, in part because strong stigma is no longer attached to single motherhood.

Another difference may be that today, after a boy or girl has had sex once, they might have multiple partners before they marry, at a rate higher than a half century ago.[5]

Male Fear Motivates the Compulsion to Control Women

Many of the abnormalities that occur around sex result from fears that men have about losing their control over women. Appalling practices such as circumcision of the clitoris or other female sexual organs, inflicted upon an estimated 130 million girls and women on this planet, result from that warped compulsion to control women's sex drives and their sexual experiences.

Evidence of female circumcision has been found in five-thousand-year-old Egyptian mummies, so we know the male compulsion to control female sexuality is an ancient and routine attitude. It persisted in other forms as well, such as the metal rings inserted into women's labia by the ancient Romans and the chastity belts (men held the keys) forced upon women during medieval times in Europe.

Clitoridectomy (the complete surgical removal of the clitoris) was even commonly practiced by physicians in nineteenth-century Britain to "treat" women found to be masturbating, a sexual release that was feared to cause insanity, but only in women. By contrast, males caught masturbating were simply told they would go to hell. Thankfully, female genital mutilation was finally outlawed in 1985 throughout Britain.

These and other, similar antifemale sexual control practices have been documented as being historically condoned by most of the world's major religions: Christianity, Judaism, Islam, and Hinduism.

Today we still see evidence of these toxic attitudes about the female sex drive forming at early ages and in seemingly innocuous ways. As a young boy, I (Brian) never had sex, but there was peer pressure to say that I had. I knew there was a sexual word (*sperm*) that sounded like *firm*, so to impress the other boys, I told them that "my firm went into her."

An older boy replied, "What do you mean, 'your firm'?"

"You know, the firm. Mine went into her."

The older boy snickered. "Then she must have been a whore."

The message that came across, even at that early age, was that any girl who had sex with you was a whore. For some males, that attitude doesn't really change, even when they become middle-aged. If females express themselves sexually, they are looked down upon, whereas men judge themselves and one another by a different standard. To "conquer" a girl or woman is seen as the male prerogative and celebrated as a rite of passage. The message that men should treat females as degraded sex objects finds widespread acceptance today, most flagrantly in the culture of rap music lyrics and videos.

When we were growing up in the 1950s and '60s, girls who had a reputation for being sexually active, whether they truly were or not, were never taken seriously either by boys or by other girls. They were treated as lepers. Imagine how that shoddy treatment shaped their self-image and sexuality later in life.

Sexual roles remain unequal between men and women in many parts of the world. Why can't a woman in the twenty-first century feel free to express her sexual needs just as men do, and not be judged or condemned for it? The answer remains the same: male fear of losing sexual control.

Males who are effeminate or gay, and those females who are tomboys or butch or lesbian, receive much the same treatment. During my (Brian's) parochial school days in the third and fourth grades, I was told by priests and nuns that murder is bad, and that equally bad is homosexuality. I learned that it was wrong to look at naked women or to masturbate. I had no idea I was even supposed to be looking at naked women. As soon as they told me it was a bad thing, what did I want to do? Look at those pictures, of course. Yet if you look at a picture of a naked woman when you are seven or eight years old and nothing happens, nothing is aroused, you begin to think there must be something wrong with you.

Anna Maria had a quite different upbringing around sexuality. I (Anna Maria) grew up in Sweden, a country which in the 1960s and '70s had a reputation for being more liberal, if not more permissive and promiscuous, than any other culture on the planet.

To some extent, Sweden's reputation was more myth than reality. It wasn't that we Swedes were more promiscuous than other people; it was our generally natural and uninhibited attitude toward nudity and our open discussion of sexual matters that made us seem on the cutting edge of the sexual revolution.

Because women didn't feel as oppressed in Sweden as in many other countries, we grew up knowing that we could become whatever we wanted to be in life, and that realization negated a lot of tension between men and women. Sex was always talked about in our family, and nudity was common, particularly when we swam together as a family in lakes or the ocean. I grew up free and natural and uninhibited about my body. I also had a good relationship with my father, which is important if a woman is to have good relationships with men later in life.

When I traveled in the 1970s to Germany, Switzerland, and other European countries, I did notice that these cultures (with the possible exception of Denmark) were sexually repressed compared to us Swedes. One factor may have been that Sweden had less religious oppression than these other cultures, less guilt and shame around the expression of sexual behaviors. By taking away secrecy around sex and the human body, the culture of Sweden helped to reduce warping, sickness, and guilt about sexual expression.

Misinformation (or No Information) Encourages Repression

It's not unnatural to want to have sex. In fact, it is unnatural *not* to want to have sex. It's unnatural for parents to take a puritan approach and not expose their child to sexual facts and ideas. Parents had better start talking about sex and take it out of the clouds; otherwise, mistakes and insanities about sex could enter their children's lives. Propaganda promoted by religious dogma has distorted the natural sexual expression of entire generations of people.

Some kids who grew up in the 1950s and 1960s got the story from their parents about how a stork came and dropped off babies, like Santa Claus dropping off presents. Others got a convoluted birds-and-bees talk from one parent or the other that left them puzzled over whether the story had meaning for them. But most kids got no information at all from their parents about sex, and, like private investigators, they had to find out for themselves by experimentation or by listening to rumors spread by friends and siblings. This absence of open and honest conversation about sex warped intimacy and relationships in ways that in later life would balloon the rates of divorce.

The sexual revolution of the 1960s rocked and rolled an entire generation's attitudes toward what was personally permissible or socially acceptable. For many U.S. teenagers of that era, a kind of schizophrenia emerged around sex and the healthy expression of the libido, as they struggled to reconcile a spirit of "free love" with the often repressive indoctrination they had received from parents and their religious and social institutions.

During our interviews for this book with veterans of that turbulent period, we noted some recurring patterns that would shape their lifelong intimate relationships. First, religious upbringing, reinforced by parental authority, proved to be the thousand-pound gorilla in the sex lives of many baby boomers.

Consider what Andrew, Reba, and Michelle told us. Andrew grew up in Chicago in a Catholic family where sex was almost never discussed. His father had made a "valiant effort," as Andrew put it, when he was fourteen years old, using birds-and-bees terminology that made Andrew laugh. "I had an understanding that marriage was a prerequisite to intimacy," Andrew related. "After having a few sexual experiences as a teenager and young adult, I developed a more Christian mind-set. [Starting] in my thirties, I practiced celibacy for fifteen years. Then I concluded that man, not God, had put these constraints on me and anyone with that point of view. But I'm still not into promiscuity. I don't feel comfortable with sex that has no intimacy. I'm now fifty-three years old and I've never been married, nor do I currently have an intimate partner."

Reba spent most of her life in Florida and had a loving, affectionate, "touchy-feely" family upbringing. "But Catholicism was my big hang-up, and it kept me a virgin until I met my husband," she explained. "I wasn't truly prepared for the sexual act itself. I was naïve about sex. Religion was like a shadow hanging over my sex life. I believed that I would make God sad if I wasn't a good girl until I married. While I've outgrown some of that, I still feel very moral about sex. It's supposed to be special and sacred. Maybe that's why I've only slept with one man in my entire life: my husband."

Michelle comes from Montreal, Canada, and had happy and loving parents, though sex was a taboo subject in their household. "The '60s sexual revolution left me with a tremendous amount of guilt. It was like I had two personalities. One was that sex outside marriage was a sin. The other was an 'anything goes' attitude of sexual freedom. That split gave me a warped view of relationships. I decided that I should marry my best friend, so I did, and there was little sexual passion in our relationship. I met my second husband at my place of employment while I was still married to my first husband. I knew I had found my soulmate. I've been married twenty-six years to my second husband. Our passion has always been based on love and intimacy."

Probably no category of teenagers from the '60s (or since) had to overcome more social stigmas, or shed more psychological conditioning, than those who discovered they were attracted to members of their own sex. A couple in their late fifties whom we know, Susan and Caroline, provide an illustration of what had to be overcome. Both grew up in New York, but they would lead separate yet similar lives until they met in Florida and became a couple just a few years ago.

Susan's parents were affectionate but not open about discussing sex or sexuality with her. The same can be said for Caroline's family. Susan looked up dirty words in the dictionary as part of her learning process, and had boyfriends she enjoyed kissing while in the fifth and sixth grades. Caroline educated herself about sex at the age of eleven by pulling the Kinsey Report on sex from under her parents' bed and by happening across a book on homosexuality called *The 10th Man*. When Caroline had her first menstrual period, it was her older brother, not her parents, who explained the puzzling changes in her body to her.

"In college," says Susan, "I had to discard the attitude I had been brought up with that sex was bad and if I had sex with someone, I was a whore. I didn't have any conscious prohibitions against homosexuality, so when I had my first sexual experience with a woman in college, it felt right to me. When I finally did tell my mother that I was sexually attracted to other women, she asked me why I still had a diaphragm in my drawer. I explained that I had been sexually active with men, but now I realized that I prefer women. The sort of emotional baggage that lingers for me from cultural conditioning is that I still have to consciously discard the idea that someone else is responsible for my pleasure."

Caroline grew up in a home where nudity in front of family members was commonplace, but so was antipathy toward homosexuality. "It seemed like my mother hated gays. At the age of twenty-one, I thought I should sleep with a guy first to see what it was like, because I had this idea that being with a man was normal. So I did, and the very next night I slept with a woman. It was clear to me that I preferred sex with women. Now I think being with a woman is perfectly normal, and I can't imagine being sexually intimate with a man."

Susan's biggest lesson drawn from confronting sexual stereotypes has been about the difference between sex and intimacy. "There is sex from a place of animalism, and there is intimacy out of choice and out of desire. I've experienced both in my life. I prefer the sex that occurs out of choice. Each has a different language. Lustful sex is fun, but intimate sex is all about the expression of profound joy."

For anyone reading this who still believes that it is unnatural or abnormal for any segment of humankind to be homosexual, consider the findings of genetically predisposed homosexual behavior within the animal kingdom. Up to fifteen hundred species of wild and captive animals have been documented as being naturally bisexual, engaging in sexual activities with their own sex and the opposite sex with equal abandon. A fascinating article in *Scientific American Mind* details how one such animal, a close relative of the chimpanzee called the bonobo, is a highly promiscuous species whose females engage in genital-to-genital rubbing of their clitorises and whose males perform oral sex on one another.[6]

Although we humans may think of ourselves as superior to the animal kingdom because we sometimes can override our genetically programmed tendencies, being homosexual or bisexual doesn't fit that pattern of self-control, as many studies of homosexuals who tried to "go straight" have demonstrated. It's absurd and sad that some religious and political groups advocate and practice attempts to "deprogram" gays and bisexuals using psychological conditioning. Any attempts they can point to as being successful probably involved either people who weren't carrying a genetic predisposition to being gay or bisexual, or those who repressed their urges in an attempt to appear heterosexual. Homosexuality is a sexual expression that rarely involves choice and is usually determined by genetics. But even if it were a matter of choice, why should anyone care about which nonviolent sexual acts consenting adults do with each other?

Stigmas around Age and Sexuality

For most of us, as children and teenagers, it was unthinkable to imagine our parents having sex. That's a common reaction. Most people, even as adults, seem to feel discomfort when it comes to thinking about their own parents having sex at any age.

Today, girls start menstruating as young as nine years old, and unless an adult fills them in on accurate details about sex, girls can develop incorrect ideologies about it at the very time when their bodies are most receptive to sexual experiences. Unless instructions are given on natural ways to relieve sexual urges, then promiscuous intercourse, pregnancy, and exposure to diseases will be the norm for many youths.

During Bill Clinton's presidency, U.S. Surgeon General M. Joycelyn Elders, MD, was forced to resign in 1994, after just fifteen months in office, because of a firestorm of controversy after she publicly suggested that masturbation should be considered a normal and healthy way of practicing safer sex. In response to a question about safe sex, she had said that masturbation is something that perhaps should be taught. She literally lost her job for being honest and, in our opinion, for being on the right side of history.

Masturbation is certainly an act superior to having promiscuous sex. It is safer, with no chance of pregnancy or of contracting diseases. It also prepares us to have satisfying intimacy as we get older, because we come to know our bodies better and learn how to give and receive pleasure. Yet masturbation is portrayed by reactionary minds and reactionary institutions as a shameful, degrading, selfish, and immature act. That is the state of mind that views sex as good only when it's done for procreation.

In parochial school, I (Brian) was indoctrinated with the belief that I would go blind if I masturbated. Every time I did, I made sure that I read something immediately afterward, anything I could get my eyes on, just to make certain that I could still see. The same people told me that if I kissed a girl of another religion, the earth would open up and I would burn in hell. So the first time I did kiss a girl of another religion, I kept one eye open to watch the ground below. Other people told me that I would get warts on my hands from masturbating. I even knew kids whose fathers would periodically check their hands for warts, and if they had one, their fathers would punish them for masturbating.

No wonder entire cultures distort the subject of sex. No wonder abominations occur in which repressed sexuality erupts into violence, rape, and molestation.

Repression Produces Strange Behaviors

Sexual orientation should be a nonissue as long as no one is harming anyone else. As long as bisexuals, homosexuals, and heterosexuals are comfortable with their sexual identity, why isn't that identity considered normal? Simply because of fear.

Evidence is emerging that human beings are predominantly, but not exclusively, of one sexual orientation or another. Yet we all have some degree of repressed bisexuality within us. In expression of sexual preferences, it all comes down to self-esteem. How much do you care about yourself, honor yourself, and respect yourself? How conflicted are you, and what do you repress?

Context also matters. Look at what happens when heterosexual men or women are in prison. The incidence of homosexuality rises. When they walk out of prison after engaging in homosexual relations, do they automatically revert to acting as exclusive heterosexuals? Many, if not most, do.

In my late twenties, I (Brian) worked and taught in India, and observed homosexual activity going on with every boy who wasn't yet married. At first I thought I was in a country of nothing but homosexual men because everywhere I looked, boys were holding hands and kissing. A friend of mine, an Indian physician, explained that this was a cultural tradition. It was a way for boys and men to release their sexual frustration. For the most part, the day they got married, they became completely heterosexual. A few remained homosexual, but no higher a percentage did so than in any western culture.

As a measure of what repression generates, think about the religious and political leaders who fly the flag of being anti- this or that, and then get caught doing what they condemn. No healthy person who is comfortable in their heterosexuality goes out of their way to condemn homosexuality. We don't know any sane and balanced heterosexual who worries about a "threat" from homosexuals. Why would anyone be aggressively opposed to homosexuality if they didn't have those tendencies in themselves? Why has there been so much child abuse and homosexual activity, for instance, among priests in the Catholic Church?

Consider the scandals involving politicians who identified themselves as "traditional family values" conservatives. U.S. Congressman Mark Foley of Florida, chairman of the House Caucus on Missing and Exploited Children, resigned after sending sexually explicit emails to young boys who worked as pages in Congress. Senator Larry Craig of Idaho pleaded guilty to soliciting sex from an undercover male policeman in an airport bathroom, but later tried to retract his plea. Imagine how miserable someone must be to seek that kind of intimacy because he feels he can't express it otherwise.

Look at the many sexual scandals involving priests and clergymen. Televangelist Jim Bakker resigned his ministry in 1987 after an affair with his secretary. Fellow televangelist Jimmy Swaggart condemned Bakker's "sexual deviancy," but within a year Swaggart was forced to reveal publicly that he was a regular customer of prostitutes. Evangelist

Ted Haggard, president of the National Association of Evangelicals, who often preached that homosexuality was an abomination against God, was forced to resign in 2006 after admitting that he had employed male prostitutes.

If such moral conservatives don't come out of the closet about their sexual desires and break the pattern of hypocrisy, repression erupts and produces strange and embarrassing behaviors. Suppressing their sexual identity, not being able to express it in a healthy way, is most evident among those who vocalize the most repressed points of view. New York Governor Eliot Spitzer, for instance, who as that state's attorney general had aggressively prosecuted escort service owners, was forced to resign in 2008 after revelations that he had spent tens of thousands of dollars on prostitutes employed by an escort service exactly like the ones he had shut down.

In contrast to the results of repression, homosexual men and women who spend most of their lives being open and unashamed about their sexual orientation are "more active, happier, and better adjusted in later life" than those who aren't open and honest about their sexuality. That was the conclusion of a 2005 study by the International Longevity Center.[7]

Damaged attitudes around sex can verge on insanity. Our strongest desire as human beings is distorted by conditioning based on fear. This can create sick minds and even, potentially, criminal minds. You are told that something is so precious and so sacred that you cannot even think about it, much less express it, and yet if you suppress those hormones and urges long enough, rape, sexual violence, and other strange and twisted behaviors can result.

Sex that isn't clean or pure or guilt-free tends to damage people and affect them for the rest of their lives, which is another reason that we wrote this book. All of us need to take the subject out of the shadows so that our unburdened minds can assist in the process of transforming sexual energy into good health to sustain long and fulfilling lives.

As a culture, we have made some progress toward being more open about sexual subjects. If you're of the right age, you may remember *The Newlywed Game*, that popular TV game show from several decades ago, on which just-married couples were questioned separately to determine how well they really knew the likes and dislikes of their spouses. Once, in answer to the question "Where, specifically, is the weirdest place that you personally have ever gotten the urge to make whoopee?" one woman replied, without hesitation, "In the ass." Her response prompted a lot of stunned expressions and stifled laughter from the studio audience, offering a revealing benchmark by which to measure social attitudes of that time. Today the question would be more direct — "Where is the strangest place you've ever had sex?" — and though the woman's answer might still draw some laughs, it would not prompt the shocked disbelief of yesteryear. Sexual practices are coming out of the closet in this day and age in western countries, and it's about time.

Warped Attitudes Lead to Sexual Dysfunction

Medical studies have accumulated considerable evidence that shows distorted attitudes about sex, and resulting sexual inhibitions, can produce sexual performance problems for both men and women. High rates of sexual dysfunction have become a worldwide phenomenon, and while poor diets, exposure to toxic chemicals, disease, and medication side effects all play important supporting roles, the underlying cause of the problem can be traced to toxic attitudes and behaviors.

For women, sexual dysfunctions include a loss of interest in sex, problems getting sexually aroused, and an inability to achieve orgasm. For men, the conditions are primarily erectile dysfunction and premature ejaculation, though a growing number of men report having lost all interest in being sexual.

To get a grip on the depth and breadth of these dysfunctions, look at these statistics from studies recently published in the *Journal of Sexual Medicine* and similar scientific journals:

- A survey of urologists and sexual medicine experts from sixty countries estimated that overall, about 40 percent of adult women and 30 percent of adult men worldwide suffer from at least one major sexual dysfunction.

- A 2005 survey of 6,700 people across China, Taiwan, South Korea, Japan, Thailand, Singapore, Malaysia, Indonesia, and the Philippines found that 27 percent of women had lost all interest in sex and 23 percent had an inability to reach orgasm; among men, 20 percent experienced premature ejaculation and 15 percent had erectile dysfunction.

- Similar polling in 2006 among Europeans in Britain, Germany, Italy, Austria, France, and Spain detected 23 percent of men and 32 percent of women with sexual dysfunctions.

- In the United States, a study of 3,005 men and women ages fifty-seven to eighty-five discovered that half of each group reported at least one bothersome sexual problem. Once people reach seventy years of age and older, sexual dysfunctions affect four out of every five men and women, with erectile difficulties being the most common complaint among men and lack of sexual desire the most common change reported by women.[8]

It's significant and no coincidence that all these surveys found a much higher rate of sexual dysfunction among women than among men. Women have suffered more from social constraints, cultural programming, and double standards around sexual beliefs and expressions of sexual behavior than men have, and while the negative effects can show up at any stage of life, the repercussions become especially pronounced when women reach menopause.

A particularly revealing piece of evidence in this regard comes from a 2006 survey of 1,335 Swedish women, ages eighteen to seventy-four years, in which it was found that narrow attitudes about sex are a good indicator of sexual dysfunction. "Likely protectors of good orgasmic function," reads the *Journal of Sexual Medicine* study, "mainly against manifest dysfunction, were: a relatively early age at first orgasm, a relatively greater repertoire of techniques used…, attaching importance to sexuality and being relatively easily sexually aroused."[9]

All the preceding attributes and experiences require a somewhat open mind, free of the influences of sexually repressive dogma. Though Sweden has had a worldwide reputation, at least since the 1960s, of being more open-minded about sex than most other countries, this study found a generation gap in how Swedish women experience their sexuality. Older women, who grew up in a less permissive environment, tended to have more sexual dysfunctions than women who were a product of more recent cultural changes. A 2005–06 report, *Ageism in America*, by the International Longevity Center in New York City, affiliated with the Mount Sinai School of Medicine, comes to this stark conclusion about the impact of cultural attitudes on sexuality: "A frank, evidence-based, constructive consideration of the meaning and importance of sexuality for health, quality of life, and the human experience is lacking.…absence of knowledge and censorship of discussion or inquiry about human sexuality result in, at best, unnecessary anxiety and confusion, and, at worst, suffering, disease, ignorance, and dysfunction."[10]

As a practical matter, one of the best indicators that negative or narrow attitudes and beliefs about sex undermine sexual performance is the success of cognitive behavioral therapy (CBT) in treating men with erectile dysfunction and women with problems experiencing orgasm. This treatment is especially important to women because not a single pharmaceutical drug or natural remedy anywhere has been shown to be beneficial for relieving orgasmic dysfunction.

Cognitive behavioral therapy is based on the idea that your thoughts can either enhance or obstruct your ability to heal, and that you can change your thoughts and their underlying toxic beliefs so that your mind can improve your health. If you believe that your genes determine your destiny and that you can't fight a disease or illness, for instance, or if you believe your emotions stand in the way of achieving wellness, this self-treatment practice can help you to remove these self-created barriers to the effective healing of many cases of sexual dysfunction.

Our core beliefs are often formed in childhood and contribute to "automatic thoughts" that influence our behaviors later in life. The first step in the cognitive behavioral process is to identify negative or irrational beliefs, and then to begin reframing or reinterpreting them in a healthier light to develop coping strategies that will be effective when the thoughts or reactions emerge again.

It's an ideal way to harness your body's own healing wisdom, and it's a technique that medical studies have shown to be effective in treating rheumatic diseases, insomnia, chronic fatigue syndrome, menopausal hot flashes, panic disorder, depression, cancer pain, and dozens of other maladies, including sexual dysfunctions. This process can be an important instrument in the toolbox of skills you carry in your life's journey.[11] Below we describe it in greater detail, with a self-help exercise for you to perform.

EXERCISE: DEPROGRAM TOXIC ATTITUDES

Cognitive behavioral therapy (CBT) is a widely used and easy-to-learn technique for treating stress, anxiety, and a variety of ailments. Basically, CBT is based on the idea that how you think about something affects how you feel and how you behave. Once you become aware of how a narrow perspective or limiting thoughts are negatively affecting you, you can find more adaptive thoughts that produce a different positive feeling about a particular situation and, with it, a different behavior. CBT has a proven track record of success, especially when combined with massage, exercise, and meditation. You can also use this technique to help identify and resolve toxic thinking styles, attitudes, and beliefs that limit your sexual satisfaction and potential.

Through this exercise, you will learn how to identify the patterns of thoughts that lead you down the paths of dysfunction, such as when you always expect the worst to happen, or when you engage in all-or-nothing thinking. Then you will learn to substitute realistic, practical, and positive thoughts in place of the toxic ones. As you go through this process, you will write new, broader mental scripts, along with an action plan, that will help you to create healthy behavioral changes.

While it is most beneficial to do cognitive therapy with a professional counselor or therapist, so that an expert can guide you through its various steps and offer his or her analysis, you can also practice this technique on your own to begin developing your action plan for attitude change.

Scenario

As an example of how the process works in practice, let's say you have a revulsion to or reluctance about performing or receiving oral sex. As long as you can remember, oral sex has been something that you have avoided and refused to engage in, or else you have performed it only after feeling pressure from your partner. You want to liberate yourself from this attitude.

Work the Problem

To begin, take a blank sheet of paper and turn it horizontally. Draw lines to create four columns on the page. Label the columns, starting from the far left side as follows:

At the top of the first column, write *Situation and Emotions*.
At the top of the second column, write *Limiting Thoughts*.
At the top of the third column, write *Styles of Thinking*.
At the top of the fourth column, write *Balanced View*.

You will work through the columns from the left to the right. First, in the left-hand column, you'll want to summarize the situation in one concise sentence, such as "My partner enjoys oral sex but I'm having a hard time with it, and I freeze up whenever this occurs." Now write down all the emotions that come up in connection with this situation, such as sadness, disgust, anger, fear, shame, guilt, helplessness, and so forth. If you're not sure what the feelings are, you might try to close your eyes and picture the situation. Take a couple of calming breaths as you do this. Notice whatever you are feeling as you recall the situation. Be as honest as you can, and write down as many emotions as you can. Remember that there is nothing wrong with your feelings, and it is okay to acknowledge them.

Now move to column two, *Limiting Thoughts*. These are the thoughts that seem to automatically arise by themselves. Often, they are related to the emotions that you just wrote down in column one. Right now, see if you can think of a statement or thought that is connected to one of your emotions. For instance, a feeling of shame might be connected to the thought "I believe oral sex is immoral." The emotion of fear or anxiety might be associated with a limiting thought such as "I worry I'll get a disease and be punished for having oral sex." You might even think about when you first had these thoughts and where this programming came from, and how this belief distorts your prospect of having a pleasurable experience with oral sex. Usually, limiting thoughts, or a narrow perspective, are fairly easy to think of and write down. Try to write at least one limiting thought for each emotion that you have identified.

Now that you have described your automatic or limiting thoughts, it is time to analyze them in column three. While thoughts in our heads may seem very real and believable, it is possible that they are not facts — but are actually cognitive distortions or thinking errors. There are eight toxic thinking patterns that most of us engage in on a daily basis, usually without being aware that they may be totally inaccurate and producing emotional unhappiness.

These eight patterns of thought are listed on pages 30–31. As you look through this list, you may notice that each of the limiting thoughts you wrote in column two matches up with a particular thinking style. The limiting statement "I worry I'll get a disease and be punished for having oral sex," mentioned above, fits the thinking style of expecting negative things to happen, or forecasting bad news. When you find the appropriate thinking style for each of the limiting thoughts in column two, write this down in column three, directly opposite the limiting thought.

1. You overgeneralize: This happens when you allow a single negative event or situation to color your perceptions. For example, "My first experience with oral sex was repugnant; therefore all oral sex will be repugnant," or "I had trouble performing oral sex well, so I quit trying to be proficient at it."

2. You engage in all-or-nothing thinking: You believe that you are either perfect or worthless at doing something. For example, "I can never orally please a partner because I'm just no good at it."

3. You often focus on the negative: Your mind gravitates toward the negative rather than the positive. For example, "My first experience with oral sex was awful, so all future experiences will be."

4. You engage in mind reading: You assume that you know what the other person is thinking without verifying that assumption. For example, "I know my partner thinks my oral sex skills are poor."

5. You engage in self-blame: You tend to assume personal responsibility for negative events when there is no reason to do so. For example, "I am at fault when my partner doesn't feel pleasure."

6. You project emotional reasoning: This means that you believe that people and situations are always a reflection of you; everything around you exists in the way that you feel about it. For example, "I feel that I am bad at giving oral sex; therefore my partner feels the same way."

7. You always expect negative things to happen: You anticipate the

worst possible outcome in any situation you confront. For example, "I know my partner will ask for oral sex and I will fail to please her [or him]."

8. You use lots of "should" statements: You have inflexible rules about how you and other people should act. For example, "I should reject oral sex because it is immoral."

Don't feel bad about having a particular thinking style. That would just be another example of the self-blame thinking style! The point here is to learn that thoughts are not necessarily facts. Be patient as you identify your thinking styles. You have taken an important step toward challenging your cognitive errors.

Create a More Balanced View

Finally, in the right-hand column, under *Balanced View*, write a series of positive responses you might cultivate to replace the limiting or self-defeating thoughts. For instance, if your mind says, "Oral sex is unclean," write, "Oral sex *can* be clean." The balanced view does not, however, need to be an exact opposite of the limiting thought. All that's necessary is for you to find a challenging statement that has some truth for you. This can be based on evidence from your own life or from the medical establishment about the safety of oral sex. Create a positive response for every negative belief or emotion, and a new, more positive belief as an alternative to the self-defeating belief. A balanced view can also be an action plan, a way for you to take steps, even small ones, toward your goal. This could include doing relaxation practices before sex, or even accepting that you may experience some fear as you go through the process of relearning how you think about this.

This process will take practice. But every time you find your mind reverting to negative beliefs about oral sex, substitute the positive beliefs as a counterbalance. Repeating this practice over time can change your core beliefs and patterns of thought. Keep in mind that CBT can be useful in addressing most any sexual dysfunction or anxiety around that dysfunction, so don't hesitate to incorporate the process into your life.

Imagine Your Sexuality

As selfishness and complaint pervert and cloud the mind,
so love with its joy clears and sharpens the vision.

— Helen Keller (1880–1968)

Desire Starts in Your Mind

To liberate the free attention necessary for developing an enduring and satisfying sex life, you must first banish anxiety, shame, guilt, and inhibitions about sexual expression. That means opening your mind to new ways of thinking about sexuality. "Sex is first and foremost a psychological issue," affirms Barnaby Barratt, PhD, president of the American Association of Sex Educators.[1]

Not only does our mind directly influence our ability to feel desire and then to achieve orgasmic pleasure, but it — and the intention we set with it — also can literally reprogram groups of cells in our body to alter their expression and function. As an illustration of this mind-over-matter power, consider the evidence presented in an article in *Scientific American Mind*, which begins with this description of a remarkable experiment:

She did not often have such strong emotions. But she suddenly felt powerless against her passion and the desire to throw herself into the arms of the cousin whom she saw at a family funeral. "It can only be because of that patch," said Marianne, a participant in a multinational trial of a testosterone patch designed to treat hypoactive sexual desire disorder, in which a woman is devoid of libido. Testosterone, a hormone ordinarily produced by the ovaries in women, is linked to female sexual function, and the women in this 2005 study had undergone operations to remove their ovaries.

After 12 weeks of the trial, Marianne had felt her sexual desire return. Touching herself unleashed erotic sensations and vivid sexual fantasies. Eventually she could make love to her husband again and experienced an orgasm for the first time in almost three years. But that improvement was not because of testosterone, it turned out. Marianne was among the half of the women who had received a placebo patch — with no testosterone in it at all.[2]

Imagine that! This woman and others in the same study had overcome biological impediments to feeling desire and even a physical inability to achieve orgasm simply by believing that the placebo they were taking was something that would heal them. What this article neglected to relate were other, equally revealing results from the study that should challenge any doubts you might have about the capacity of your mind to dramatically alter your physical reality.

Here is the background. To be eligible for participation in this study, which was conducted over a twenty-four-week period at clinics in the United States, Canada, and Australia, women had to be between twenty-six and seventy years of age and had to report having had a satisfactory sex life before surgery (a hysterectomy and removal of their ovaries) destroyed their sexual desire and their ability to have an orgasm.

Participants were equally and randomly divided into two groups: one who wore testosterone patches on their abdomens, and a second group who wore placebo patches (with no active ingredient) on their abdomens. None of the women knew which group she was in, and each woman kept a weekly sexual activity diary. As the researchers evaluated the contents of these weekly diaries, they took note of any adverse reactions being reported and, if necessary, placed the study participant under medical supervision. Adverse reactions were defined as acne or similar skin eruptions, unwanted hair growth, or a deepening of the voice, all conditions consistent with the body's overreaction to testosterone.

Most people might suspect that these adverse physical reactions to testosterone would be restricted to the group actually receiving the testosterone treatment. But the powers of the human mind do not always conform to the self-limiting boundaries of our low expectations. Twenty-two women were forced to discontinue their participation in the study due to adverse reactions, and of those, thirteen were in the placebo group!

By every adverse-event measure for women who completed the study trial, researchers found the placebo group either equaled or exceeded the testosterone group:

- Acne outbreaks: seventeen from the placebo group; seventeen from the testosterone group
- Unwanted hair growth: eighteen from the placebo group; sixteen from the testosterone group
- Voice deepening: eight from the placebo group; seven from the testosterone group

What further confounded the expectations of the medical researchers was the finding that in nearly every category of sexual functioning — arousal, orgasm, pleasure, responsiveness — the placebo group reported significant improvements that rivaled those of the treatment group at the end of the twenty-four weeks.

Writing in the *Journal of Clinical Endocrinology & Metabolism*, the thirteen study authors tried to explain their findings this way: "The placebo response in this study is consistent with that in other reports related to sexual functioning. All women enrolled in our study stated at baseline that they desired an improvement in their sex lives, and participating in the study may have increased dialogue regarding sexual satisfaction between the study subjects and their partners."[3]

Since a reference was made to "other reports" with similar results, it would be instructive to sketch the findings of a second testosterone/placebo study from 2000, reported in the *New England Journal of Medicine*. A group of seventy-five women, ages thirty-one to fifty-six, went through a three-stage clinical trial to test whether their sexual functioning could be improved in the wake of hysterectomies and surgery that removed their ovaries. In the first stage, lasting twelve weeks, the women wore placebo patches on their abdomens; in the second and third stages, they wore testosterone patches, with the third stage delivering twice as much testosterone into their bodies as the second stage. All the stages occurred in random-order assignments, so the women never knew when they were wearing the placebo patch.

In premenopausal women, about half the natural production of testosterone occurs in the ovaries (the other half comes from the adrenal glands), but if their ovaries are removed, their serum testosterone level can drop by up to 80 percent. This study found that when the participants were wearing the placebo patch, their testosterone levels increased to measures equal to those found in the second stage of testosterone treatment, but were not as high as during the more powerful dosages of testosterone in stage three.

What was most extraordinary was the finding that women under the age of forty-eight, while on the placebo, increased their testosterone production to a near-normal range, yet, as the study authors noted, "there was no further improvement during testosterone treatment." In other words, the mind power of positive expectations alone healed most of the women in the placebo group by somehow enabling them to naturally produce higher levels of testosterone, presumably from the adrenal glands, to compensate for the loss of their ovaries.

Another measure used by the researchers to assess sexual recovery was the frequency of sexual intercourse during the study. Women in the placebo stage of the trial increased their weekly number of sexual encounters at the same rate as those in the stage one testosterone group. In every other category measured — thoughts of desire, arousal, orgasmic pleasure, and relationship satisfaction — the placebo stage participants experienced significant improvements compared to how they had rated their sexual lives before the study began.

"We can only speculate as to the origin of the strong placebo response in our study, why it was greater in the younger women, and why it tended to mask further effects of testosterone," observed the twelve researchers who conducted this experiment.[4]

The implications of these two medical studies should be underlined. Open and honest sexual dialogue between intimate partners intensifies desire, satisfaction, and physical functioning. But, more important, when you join a positive expectation with an intention that you set either consciously or unconsciously, you create a dynamic synergy that can be channeled for your own self-transformation. It can literally change your body and your life.

Keep a Sexually Active Mind

Cells affect the mind and the mind affects the cells in our body. As evidence for this statement, consider wet dreams. They're called nocturnal emissions, which sounds a little like a trip into space. But a wet dream is purely a hormonal activation that creates imagery in the mind. The body is crying out, saying, "Please utilize and express this energy." The cells of the mind are responding to the sex hormone messages of the body, and this creates sex imagery in the dream imagination, complete with a physical release. The biology of the human body encodes imagery into the brain, and this can be a tool for healing, once you learn how to master guided-imagery techniques.

The placebo effect is a psychological component of many aphrodisiacs, and it gives users the sensation that the aphrodisiac is effective. Some people feel more sexually vital simply because they believe the aphrodisiac will work. The placebo effect is also seen in negative sexual expectations — if you fear you'll have arousal problems, you probably will. The same principle is at work in disease and the healing process. People must be convinced that they have a reason to stay alive. People hold on to their pride, if they want to survive, and such people have a much higher recovery rate than those who choose to believe the disease will kill them.

Our sex drive helps to keep us vital, which in turn extends our life span. A mature and healthy relationship involves both partners openly sharing about who they're attracted to and why. That's part of the spark of life. You can share these fantasies with each other without necessarily having to act them out.

Former President Jimmy Carter talked about having lust in his heart in that famous *Playboy* magazine interview in the 1970s. He had the courage to be truthful. It was a healthy thing to say because it would have been a lie for him or for any of us to say that we don't ever lust after people other than our intimate partner or spouse. Women are just as interested in looking at men as men are in looking at women. What's unhealthy is to think that you shouldn't look. Such denial warps people.

We should be flirting until the day we die at 120 years of age. We should remain constantly interested in sexuality at some level throughout our life. The way we handle the subject of sex is criminal, especially in educating young people. We've made sex so taboo that it shouldn't be discussed, yet we think about it constantly, so why shouldn't we discuss it?

We're not suggesting that sex should be promiscuous or involve senseless risk-taking. How many hollow sexual encounters have you had in your life that made you feel worse afterward? Every action that serves the sexual impulse needs to be one of integrity, or we create conflicts for ourselves that will undermine the health-positive effects of sexual activity. If an overly active sex drive becomes impulsive and a person acts out such impulses in a mindless way, they engage in an untamed hormonal process that abuses a gift of nature.

Many hundreds of people we've worked with over the years have struggled with the repercussions of having grown up in homes where parents didn't express intimacy to each other, or even express love to their children. These are traumas in the making. By the age of six, these children had developed the impression that normal relationships don't involve touching or healthy physical contact. How do we break that cycle? It starts in your mind.

Sexual nutrition of the mind is a type of sustenance we can't always measure as we do nutrients. Yet sexual interest is a lifelong preoccupation. Young children primp before mirrors, just as the elderly do. Children in puberty ask one another, "Did he [or she] like me?" The same conversations can occur in nursing homes. We all need to feel sexually desirable. The only people who don't seem to act out this need are some of the mentally ill, who often totally lose interest in making themselves sexually attractive.

Imagination plays a vital role in keeping your sex drive humming. An imaginary experience — whether it is a wet dream, or seeing a film or a picture, or even witnessing other people being intimate — is usually the first time that our sexual desire is stimulated. There's a lot of religiously driven ignorance behind attempts to suppress these early natural thoughts. We know a woman whose father told her, as she was growing up, that she should never initiate sex with a man; only men were supposed to initiate sex. If she did, she would go to hell. That sort of toxic conditioning can take a lifetime to overcome.

As young children, we aren't sexual, but we're naturally inquisitive. Later the hormones kick in, sexuality arises, and we're off experimenting. Because of all the artificial hormones in the environment, puberty now starts at much younger ages than ever before. Menarche used to be common at twelve to fourteen years of age. Now it often occurs at eight to ten years of age. It's also more common to hear of young boys prematurely developing deep voices and facial hair. These physiological changes occurring throughout an entire generation further complicate our attempts to manage sexual expression in a healthy way.

If people freed themselves of preconceived notions about sexuality and aging and embraced sex as a vital force, a force as important as the food we eat and the spiritual faith we hold, we might attain a culture that's psychologically healthy about the expression of sexuality.

Women Can Have Wet Dreams, and Ejaculate, Too!

It's well known that males experience wet dreams during their sleep. This release of sex hormones, which inspires sexual imagery, usually begins prior to puberty and, depending on masturbation habits, can extend through the teenage years and even into adulthood. According to research by sexologist Alfred Kinsey, 83 percent of men experience nocturnal emissions at some point in their lives. In cultures where masturbation is actively suppressed, that figure approaches 100 percent.

Less well studied is the female version of the wet dream, which involves vaginal fluid secretions accompanied by stimulating erotic imagery in the mind. A survey of 5,628 women in the United States conducted by Kinsey in 1953 found that about 40 percent of these women had experienced orgasms in their sleep.[5]

In many countries, up through the nineteenth century, a male reporting nocturnal emissions was diagnosed as having a "disease" called spermatorrhoea, or seminal weakness. Treatments that included castration were often undertaken. Women who reported sexual arousal during their sleep were thought to have been visited by incubi, defined as demons by the Church, and they sometimes were subjected to exorcisms.

Today, we know that nocturnal emissions in both males and females are nature's way of announcing the body's sexual need to express itself. Put another way, it's God's way of saying, "I'm going to clean your pipes if you don't do it on your own."

Sexual arousal and climax in men and women share many physiological features. Both the penis and clitoris become erect from arterial blood flow stimulated by arousing thoughts or physical manipulation.

Orgasm for both sexes results in the sudden release of the hormone oxytocin from the pituitary gland.

Men don't have a monopoly on ejaculation at orgasm. According to *The Sexual Brain*, by biology professor Simon LeVay, about 40 percent of women emit a spurt of glandular fluid at climax.[6] The fluid is produced by glands near the urethra that may be comparable to the male prostate gland. These emissions occur most commonly during vaginal or anal intercourse, rather than from direct stimulation of the clitoris.

Want to Implant a "Sex Chip" in Your Brain?

Some old movies can give us a hint of what is to come. In 1968, the Jane Fonda film *Barbarella* featured an orgasm-producing device, as did the 1973 Woody Allen film *Sleeper*, which called its sex stimulator an Orgasmatron.

If your imagination no longer supports your sexual excitement and sexual expression, some scientists recommend that you be implanted with an electronic "sex chip" to directly stimulate the pleasure centers of your brain to facilitate orgasms.

A 2007 article in *Nature Reviews Neuroscience* features two British scientists predicting that within a decade there would be scientific breakthroughs enabling the development of such chips, which can compensate for a low libido with deep brain stimulation.[7] Similar technology has already been used to treat Parkinson's disease.

"There is evidence that this chip will work," Tipu Aziz, a professor of neurosurgery at John Radcliffe hospital in Oxford, told the *Sunday Times* of London. "A few years ago a scientist implanted such a device into the brain of a woman with a low sex drive and turned her into a very sexually active woman. She didn't like the sudden change, so the wiring in her head was removed."[8]

Visualize Your Sexual Potential

Your own imagination can be harnessed to transform yourself. Guided imagery is a healing technique that can benefit your mind, body, and spirit. Numerous medical studies have shown it to be beneficial in managing stress, anxiety, depression, and pain. You can also use it to summon the powers of imagination to envision and then fulfill your sexual potential.

Like most people, you have probably become physically aroused by a sexual fantasy, which is a form of visualization or guided imagery. This technique can be used to literally redefine the shape, size, and strength of our bodies. To some extent, the link between our thoughts and body chemistry relies upon the powerful placebo effect, which anyone can learn to harness using visualization exercises. Simple guided-imagery exercises can be used to improve your sexual vitality and performance, as we will explain later in this chapter.

Many ancient cultures traditionally used visualization and guided imagery in their healing rituals to produce desired physical responses. Medical researchers now suspect these beneficial responses are closely related to the placebo effect, in which our beliefs bring about cellular and chemical changes in the body.

Techniques for harnessing the healing power of imagination are widely taught today. Guided imagery differs from visualization in one important respect: visualization involves only the use of mental images, whereas guided imagery draws upon four of the senses: sight, smell, taste, and hearing.

Scientific support for the effectiveness of guided imagery in altering the body comes from many sources. Here are just a few examples from the medical literature:

- In 2004, a group of twenty-eight women suffering from osteoarthritis listened to recordings that described pleasant scenes and guided them in evoking all their senses around this imagery. After three months of these sessions, the guided-imagery group experienced significant reductions in pain and increased mobility, compared to a control group who received no guided-imagery training. Carol Baird, associate professor of nursing at Purdue University, a coauthor of the study, concluded that guided imagery is easy to use, inexpensive, and suitable for self-care.

- An American Cancer Society review of guided-imagery studies from 1966 to 1998 found the technique effective in the treatment of pain, depression, anxiety, stress, and the side effects of chemotherapy. These "focused daydreams," as some practitioners refer to the technique, affect the endocrine, nervous, and immune systems, perhaps because imagery is akin to a primary language of the human body.

- You can even burn calories simply by imagining yourself doing it. A study published in *Psychological Science* in 2007 evaluated eighty-four female room attendants at seven hotels. One group was told that cleaning rooms is good exercise, and they were given specific examples of how their duties burned calories. Subjects in the control group were not given this information. Four weeks later, the group who believed they were burning more calories was found to have a decrease in weight, blood pressure, body fat, waist-to-hip ratio, and body mass index compared to the control group. The results support the idea that exercise affects health in part via the placebo effect.

- The most revealing study of all documenting these mind-over-matter effects was conducted in 2007 at Bishop's University in Quebec, Canada. Thirty male university athletes were divided into three groups to measure guided imagery's effects on their strength and fitness. The first group did nothing outside their usual exercise routine, while the second group went through two weeks of highly focused strength training for one specific muscle. The third group, the experimental group, did nothing more than listen to audio CDs that guided them in imagining that they were going through the same workout as group two, the exercise group.

Results from this study were startling, to say the least. Group one participants, who did only their normal routines, saw no gains in muscle strength, a finding that surprised no one. Group two, the muscle exercisers, saw a 28 percent gain in strength. But group three, those who just imagined themselves exercising, actually experienced a 24 percent gain in muscle strength, almost as much as the exercisers.

Consider the possible implications of this study. It might well be that some women could grow larger breasts simply by using guided-imagery techniques. The possibilities are end-less, and it's a fertile ground for future scientific studies.[9]

You need an open mind to make guided imagery consistently work for you. Children are especially skilled at using this technique because they have an easier time believing new ideas, and possess fewer preconceived notions and less cynicism than most adults.

But everyone is capable of mastering the technique, as evidenced by how naturally a sexual fantasy proves arousing, causing erections in men and vaginal wetness in women. This is the most direct experience of imagery and imagination that most of us have.

Guided imagery is a power that can be directed to address sexual dysfunctions, to supercharge your sexual vitality, and to heighten your response to a sexual partner. See the exercise at the end of this chapter to get started.

Beware: Toxic Sex Can Be Addictive

While many people complain about experiencing impotence or a lack of sexual desire, some men and women are never able to fully satisfy their lust because for them, sex is an addiction. It's a preoccupation that starts in the brain — some study evidence indicates a possible genetic predisposition — and it filters through the imagination until obsessive-compulsive sexual imagery and thoughts about sexual activities dominate a person's life.

Compulsive sexual behavior is often as devastating to self-esteem and personal relationships as compulsive gambling, alcoholism, or drug addiction. Despite what many sex addicts may say they feel during the throes of passion, therapists claim that most of them aren't really enjoying the sexual act, either alone or with others, because sex is just a way for them to numb painful feelings, to stop feeling lonely, or to simply pass the time when they're bored.

With more widespread access to Internet pornography over the past few years, sex addiction has become "gender neutral," reports psychologist Mark Schwartz, former director of the Masters and Johnson Institute in St. Louis.[10] Female sex addicts formerly acted out their compulsions by having affairs or even becoming prostitutes, but many now develop and express their sexual obsessions through online cybersex conversations with strangers, or by watching pornographic movies online and on DVDs.

Mayo Clinic psychologists estimate that up to 6 percent of U.S. adults experience some form of addiction to sexual activity, which could translate into as many as 10 million people.[11] One indicator of the problem's reach might be the explosive growth in the number of Sexaholics Anonymous and Sex Addicts Anonymous chapters, with all fifty states, most large cities, and many nations of the world hosting these groups, whose programs are modeled after the twelve-step structure of Alcoholics Anonymous.

One-third of people seeking treatment for sex addiction are women, according to sexologists. Female sex addicts, according to many experts, generally crave intimacy and use sex to secure it, but once they are in a relationship, their fear of sustaining true intimacy compels them to abandon the relationship and move on to the next fantasy.

Both sex and love are highly addictive, if we're to believe brain scans that show sex and love activate the same brain areas as those activated by cocaine in addicts' brains. "If there is a difference between sex and love addiction, I don't know what it is," says self-confessed sex addict Susan Cheever, whose 2008 book, *Desire: Where Sex Meets Addiction*, explores the boundaries between feelings of passion and addiction. She cites a study showing that more than half of cocaine users have sexual compulsion problems. Many alcoholics also display symptoms of sex addiction once they have been treated for alcoholism, which is what happened in Cheever's case.[12]

Adultery is "the drunk driving of sex addiction": that is how Cheever describes it.[13] Problem drinkers who are also sex addicts crave the thrill of exciting and forbidden sexual encounters. Adultery is the thrill of choice for many sex addicts because it gives them the rush of a fantasy combined with experimentation.

Neuroscientists recognize that pornography also gives users a strong chemical "hit," comparable to that of a drug. Pornography stimulates the release of dopamine and serotonin, both naturally occurring brain chemicals. With enough exposure to these porn-inspired chemical hits, visual imagery can replace sex with another human being as a more satisfying type of sexual encounter, but one that can be just as toxic to relationships as adultery.

Having an interest in pornography and frequently engaging in sexual activity may not be, in and of themselves, addictions or addictive. The difference between healthy and unhealthy sexual interests can often be discerned by truthful answers to the series of questions posted on the Sexaholics Anonymous website (www.sa.org) and on another website (www.sexhelp.com) maintained by a sex psychologist.

Here are some revealing questions to ask yourself:

- Have you ever felt that maybe you can't control your sexual behavior or thoughts?
- Do you regularly use sex to relieve stress and anxiety, or to escape your problems?
- Are you rarely, if ever, satisfied by your sexual encounters?
- Are you frequently distracted from your work and from your daily activities by uncontrollable sexual thoughts and feelings?
- Though you may love your spouse and feel sexually compatible with this person, do you still masturbate regularly or seek sexual gratification outside your relationship?
- To get aroused or to reach orgasm, must you and/or your partner always "talk nasty" to each other?

If your answer was yes to two or more of these questions, you might want to explore the possibility that your sexual expression has become compulsively toxic, or may be getting unhealthier than you or your partner might want. It might be beneficial to access the websites mentioned above, as well of those of related groups, to see if help is available in your area.

How Common Is Sex Addiction?

Sex addiction expert Dr. Patrick Carnes developed a thirty-three-question sexual addiction screening test, which was used by self-described recovered sex addict Michael Leahy, author of *Porn University*, to survey 28,798 students at 110 colleges and universities in the United States and Canada during 2006–08. About 59 percent of those surveyed were male, 41 percent female.

Some of the highlights of his survey findings include:

- Between the ages of ten and fourteen, at least 69 percent of males had their first exposure to pornography; 68 percent of females had their first exposure at age thirteen or older.
- By nearly two to one (8 percent versus 5 percent), more females than males regularly sought sexual pleasure by sadomasochistically experiencing or inflicting sexual pain.
- About 5 percent of women and 13 percent of men confessed to having had sex with a minor.
- In answer to the question "Do you have trouble stopping your own inappropriate sexual behaviors?," 26 percent of males and 18 percent of females said yes.
- At least 38 percent of males and 23 percent of females said they had made unsuccessful efforts to stop engaging in sexual activities.[14]

EXERCISE: REFOCUS YOUR SEX VISION

Guided-imagery CDs are available from many sources, and they can be adapted to fit your sexual goals and needs. Meanwhile, here is an exercise that you can perform on your own.

Getting Started

Let's say you want to intensify blood flow to your genitals for greater sensitivity the next time you make love to your partner.

Find a quiet and comfortable place to sit. Close your eyes. You can play an environmental CD, one with sounds of ocean waves or a gentle wind through the trees, to accompany this "journey."

How to Do It

Focus first on your breathing. Breathe in deeply, then slowly release your breath. Do this repeatedly until you feel relaxed. Let that relaxation and a feeling of bodily softness spread from your head to your feet.

Imagine a bright white light inside your head. Visualize it spreading to each part of your body. Keep this image in your mind's eye for as long as you can.

Next, visualize your partner in the nude. Admire every part of his or her body and caress it with your mind. Let your imagination linger over this image.

Now visualize your own genitals. Feel them heating up. Imagine that you feel heat flowing from your own genitals to your partner's genitals. See this energy flow as a white light moving back and forth between the two of you until it is one continuous light.

Do this exercise twice a day for up to twenty minutes at each sitting.

When you have your next intimate encounter with your partner, it might be helpful to softly play the same environmental music in the background that you used in your practice sessions.

Express Your Sexuality

Of the delights of this world,
man cares most for sexual intercourse,
yet he has left it out of his heaven.

— Humorist Mark Twain (1835–1910)

How Experimentation Can Intensify Sexual Satisfaction

Annette and Irving met while students at Utah State University in the early 1970s and married not long afterward. Both had been members of the Mormon Church, which helped to insulate them from the sexual experimentation going on among their generational peers.

Over the next three decades, they raised three children and lived a rather mainstream middle-class life. But by their early fifties, the passion was gone from their marriage. Irving no longer had the sexual desire or potency to satisfy Annette, so she began living out her sexual fantasies on the Internet. Eventually, Irving discovered that his sexual problems were a by-product of a tumor growing on his pituitary gland. Medical treatment corrected the problem, and his libido returned to normal.

Annette's experiences of sharing sexual fantasies with other men on the Internet inspired her to suggest to her husband that they spice up their relationship by visiting a swingers' club in Portland, Oregon. "I was more ready to play with others than he was," Annette recalled. "He was reluctant at first because he didn't want to hurt our marriage. But he agreed to go one weekend. I was excited to be there and see people of all ages very free and open and expressive with their sexuality. We've been going to the club on occasion for the past three years. And, yes, we always practice safe sex."

Though Annette doesn't necessarily think this lifestyle would work for many long-married couples, she and Irving do believe it has strengthened their marriage in numerous ways. Jealousy inevitably surfaced in the beginning, when they saw each other flirting or having sex with other people. But they talked their way through these feelings of insecurity and, in the process, deepened their understanding and appreciation of each other.

"This lifestyle has made sex between us much more exciting and rewarding. We typically make love with each other every day, sometimes twice a day. Our fantasy life is much richer now, too. We needed something to expand ourselves and grow together. We saved our marriage by doing this. These experiences have reinforced the decision I made thirty-four years ago in choosing Irving as a mate."

Opening the Pandora's box of sexual experimentation certainly isn't for everyone, especially if one or both partners are insecure about the relationship or their own sexuality. But we have known couples who have sex outside their relationship, in an honest and open way that actually strengthens their intimacy and relationship. That takes a particularly secure pair of people who completely trust and share honestly with each other.

Extramarital affairs are viewed very differently in Europe, especially France, than in the United States, and many cultures throughout the world still have a harem mentality regarding women. There are cultures in which women have more than one husband. And, of course, we still find today the American fundamentalist Mormons who engage in the practice of having multiple wives. Only on a biological basis does this seem to make sense. Why not have more seeds coming in to perpetuate the tribe and species? Some anthropologists speculate that polygamy may have been a protection mechanism to strengthen cultural cohesion.

Infidelity Is Increasing among Women

Having sex outside of marriage used to be considered a primarily male transgression, at least until the sexual revolution of the 1960s, which expanded women's attitudes about their own permissible boundaries of sexual expression.

Women have closed the adultery gap, and they have done so most quickly since 1991, a year in which about 5 percent of women over sixty years of age confessed adultery to University of Washington behavioral researchers in a nationwide survey. By 2008, that number had tripled to 15 percent of women over sixty admitting to having had adulterous affairs. For younger women, those thirty-five years old and below, about 15 percent also say they have been unfaithful to their spouses.[1]

But these numbers may be seriously understated. A 2007 study published in the *Journal of Family Psychology* reported on a survey of 4,884 married women. These survey interviews were conducted either face to face or by anonymous computer questionnaires. Just 1 percent of women in the face-to-face interviews admitted to adultery in the previous year, compared to more than 6 percent of women who admitted to it in anonymous responses.[2]

A possible answer to why many women aren't honest about adultery comes from Helen F. Fisher, research professor of anthropology at Rutgers University, who told the *New York Times*, "Men want to think women don't cheat, and women want men to think they don't cheat, and therefore the sexes have been playing a little psychological game with each other."[3]

One explanation for the increase in adulterous affairs may simply be that more couples are unhappy with each other and their marriages than ever before. Add to that a loss of respect for the institution of marriage, especially the idea of lifelong commitment, combined with more sexual temptations than ever before (via the Internet), and the ingredients are in place for some people to feel that they have license to express sexual dissatisfactions by acting out sexual fantasies.

Why Do Men Really Cheat on Their Wives?

Nearly one in three men will cheat on their wives during marriage, according to marriage counselor M. Gary Neuman, who surveyed hundreds of husbands in an attempt to understand why they're unfaithful for his 2008 book *The Truth about Cheating: Why Men Stray and What You Can Do to Prevent It.*

Despite what you might think, most men do *not* have sex outside of marriage because they find the other woman more physically attractive than their spouse. Neuman's research found that 92 percent of cheating husbands reported that the reason they strayed wasn't primarily sex, and 88 percent of those surveyed said the other woman was no better looking or in any better physical shape than their wife. "The majority said it was an emotional disconnection, specifically a sense of feeling underappreciated," Neuman concludes. "Men look strong, look powerful and capable. But on the inside they're insecure like everybody else. They're searching for somebody to build them up to make them feel valued."

A further piece of sobering news for women that emerges from Neuman's surveys is that 55 percent of the cheating husbands "have either not told their wives, or lied after being confronted with hard evidence." Just 7 percent of the cheaters ever confessed their infidelity to their wives without being asked. Most men meet the woman they have an affair with at their place of employment or through a friendship that developed while pursuing a hobby such as golf or bowling.[4]

Neuman offers six warning signs of marital infidelity:

1. **He spends more time away from home.** Most cheating men surveyed said that more time spent away from home was a sign that they were close to or already involved in infidelity. Although women can't keep tabs on a husband's whereabouts

during the workday, it still seems that cheating men find extra time to slip away from home, not just work.

2. The couple has sex infrequently. Only 43 percent of men surveyed said that frequency of sex with their wives decreased once the infidelity began. One might wonder, Why such a small number? In many struggling marriages at high risk for infidelity, couples have sex only about once every couple of months.

3. He avoids contact with his wife. The contact a woman has with her husband, even if it is about the ordinary business of life, helps the couple develop a continuing general awareness of each other. His avoidance of her calls or desire not to spend time with her points to a desire to disconnect, whether or not he is conscious of it.

4. He criticizes her more. Often, cheating men will criticize their wives seemingly out of the blue. If a woman notices her husband criticizing her for things he used to find amusing, she should keep her eyes open for other signs.

5. He starts more fights with his wife. The criticism mentioned above often leads to more fights. If a marriage becomes increasingly contentious, it may be at risk for infidelity.

6. He mentions another woman, a female "friend," in casual conversation. Most cheating occurs with friends, not in one-night stands meant just for sex. When a husband begins to talk about a woman at the office he really admires, he may be telling his wife about a real or fantasized potential mistress straight to her face.

Confidence and Self-Esteem Enhance Desirability

While we emphasize engaging in sexual activity within committed relationships, we also recognize that singles need outlets for sexual expression. We're not recommending promiscuity, yet single people may have to be self-serving at times because a great many physiological problems and illnesses are directly related to the absence of sexual activity.

We all need to stay sexually stimulated in some aspect of our lives. And self-esteem is the key to being and feeling sexually desirable. When you feel confident, what you emit hormonally from your body is very different than what you project when you're insecure. Needless to say, confident people usually attract other confident people, unless toxic character traits keep them stuck in negative patterns in which they return to the same bad relationships.

A study done at the University of Texas and published in August 2007 in the *Archives of Sexual Behavior* surveyed hundreds of college students in an attempt to determine why people have sex with each other. This may seem, at first glance, to be an easy question to answer, but the researchers came up with 237 different reasons why people choose to have sex. The most frequently mentioned reason was stress reduction; not far behind was the desire to boost one's self-esteem. The more sexual partners some students had, the more desired or loved they felt.[5]

The ultimate example of a fulfilled existence is sexual intimacy, especially when it accompanies romantic love. But unless you are fulfilled in most other areas of your life, we can assure you that you won't feel fulfilled sexually, either. If you're being intimate while thinking about how bad a day you had at work, you're burdened by a distraction unless you know how to de-stress.

A Chemical Soup Determines Attraction

Intimacy alone can't make you happy, but it's certainly an important component of happiness. Sexual fulfillment is the cherry on the cake of life. People in toxic relationships need to raise their own self-worth so they won't tolerate a relationship that drains their energy and undermines their happiness. Fix yourself first to feel sexual, confident, and desirable, and this will in turn attract to you sexually desirable partners.

We all know intuitively that a chemical bonding occurs between two people in love. Pheromones and other hormones create the chemical soup that governs the initial instinct of sexual attraction. A soulmate, in this respect, is someone who is totally symbiotic with you and harmonizes with you at the chemical level. When I (Brian) walked into the room where I met my future wife, Anna Maria, I instantly fell in love with her at some level. At the hormonal level, our soups mixed. Everyone I know in long-term intimate relationships who defines themselves and their partners as soulmates tells a similar story. They thought it was their heart speaking, when in fact it was their hormones.

A lack of intimacy often results in sadness and disease. By contrast, here at the Hippocrates Health Institute, we have routinely seen how the return of sexual intimacy to someone's life quite often facilitates a recovery from illness and disease. As we indicated in an earlier chapter, it all starts when we reach a new frontier of openness about sexual intimacy and we affirm its importance to our lives.

A man in his seventies with stage four liver cancer came to us for a consultation. He was understandably sad and distressed about the diagnostic workup that showed he was dying of this disease. All his medical reports were bleak. But when we asked him about his relationship, he glowed like a boy because he had just celebrated his fiftieth wedding anniversary. He spoke with elation about his wife and how they had known each other since childhood. As grim as his physical circumstances were, the key to his door of hope was to address that relationship. He boasted that even in the middle of chemotherapy, he continued making love to his wife. This man eventually put himself in total remission from cancer, and the reason was that he realized he wanted to stay alive to keep his intimacy with his wife. When we saw him next, after two years of remission, he told us again that he and his wife made love numerous times a week.

It would be arrogant to think that we are somehow above the instinct of sex. If you're a woman, once you're beyond childbearing age, one of the blessings of maturity and menopause is that you can still make love. Nature provided us with the ability to continue intimacy even after it no longer has any function for perpetuation of the species. The emotional and spiritual fulfillment of the sexual instinct is too often regulated away later in life by a person's belief system or by the rigidities of habituated behaviors.

It's not just us claiming that healthy sex promotes physical health. A body of medical evidence supports what we are saying. Two pioneering studies found that couples in active sexual relationships derive health benefits from loving relations because their endocrine systems harmonize, which modulates their autonomic nervous systems.[6] Still another study found that unmarried men and women who remain sexually active after the age of fifty report a much greater satisfaction with life than those over fifty who are no longer sexually active.[7]

We believe there isn't a person on the planet who doesn't want a loving partner and happiness. Even people chronically afflicted by depression and cynicism must on occasion feel glimmers of hope. What prevents love and happiness from happening is often fear: the fear that you aren't good enough, or you will screw it up, or you aren't ready for the love of your life.

If you don't have sex in a relationship, you don't have a completely intimate relationship. It's that simple. You can have all the intellectual compatibility, all the friendship you want, but if you stop making love, then the relationship suffers, and often one of you will look outside the relationship to receive the intimacy you crave. There is always an underlying volcano ready to erupt in these relationships. It may manifest as silly battles over power in the home. Rather than resolving their sexual frustration and repression, the couple may try to resolve their problems intellectually.

A committed relationship does not mean only marriage. There are other levels of committed relationships. Aging people cohabitate, often with a level of intimacy. The critical reason for sex is to perpetuate humanity, and sexuality is an instinctive drive. Regardless of one's age, when that desire is not fulfilled, the lack creates a psychological impact due as much to hormonal chemistry as to the pressures of social norms.

The more intimacy you have, the more your chemical soup blends with another's, and that creates even more potential for eroticism. Yet at the same time this potential is developing, there is a downside: what happens to the mind with prolonged familiarity, when people start feeling sex is the same old boring routine. This happens frequently with married couples. Ironically, infidelity, after its discovery and forgiveness, sometimes reactivates the passion in relationships. Below we list other steps you can take to respice your chemical soup.

Five Steps to Sexual Healing

1. Understand the chemistry of desire and where it really comes from.
2. "Feel" your way into where your images of good and bad relationships come from.
3. Learn how to let go of past good and bad experiences.
4. Develop a sexually attractive persona by becoming a healthy, vital person.
5. Allow yourself to aspire to develop a spiritual understanding of sexuality.

Harness the Healing Power of Touch

Reaching out and touching someone — and being touched — bestows tremendous health benefits. It's an energy exchange that produces biochemical enhancers for overall health.

The first concrete medical evidence for this effect came in the 1930s, when physicians noticed that certain nurseries had much higher mortality rates for newborn babies than did other nurseries. An investigation revealed that some nurseries encouraged their nursing staff to hold and cuddle newborns, which reduced mortality rates and the incidence of illness. The nurseries with the high death and illness rates did not emphasize touching as a therapy.

Ashley Montagu pointed out in his pioneering book, *Touching: The Human Significance of the Skin*, that "at Bellevue Hospital in New York, following the institution of 'mothering' on the pediatric wards, the mortality rates for infants under one year fell from 35 percent to less than

10 percent by 1938. What the child requires if they are to prosper, it was found, is to be handled and carried, caressed and cuddled, and cooed to, even if it isn't breastfed."[8]

Subsequent clinical research showed the immunologic functions of touching. In one study, ten infants were divided into two groups at ten weeks of age: a group who were touched, and a control group who were not touched. In the group whose mothers stroked their infants until six months of age, the babies had fewer colds, vomiting, and diarrhea than infants who didn't receive the touching attention.[9]

At Miami's Touch Research Institute, scientists discovered that premature infants who received at least three massages a day over five days gained 53 percent more body weight than infants who didn't receive regular touch attention.[10] For adults, touch through massage can stimulate foreplay and activate orgasmic states, while strengthening the immune systems of both partners. Regular doses of loving touch will make you healthier and happier.

Studies of people later in life uncovered evidence of "significant biochemical differences between humans who have enjoyed adequate tactile stimulation and those who have not," in Montagu's words. "Adequate mothering is necessary for the development of healthy sexual behavior." Other studies detected a pattern in which women who failed to receive adequate tactile stimulation as babies and children grew up engaging in sexual relations "in a desperate attempt to gain some contact with their own bodies."[11]

Montagu's book further documents the relation of skin and touching to all aspects of mental and physical health, especially among senior citizens, and describes how touching the skin confers more than just immunological benefits to health. "Tactile needs do not seem to change with aging — if anything, they seem to increase...when, in old age, the male's sexual capacities are diminished or completely reduced, the tactual hunger is more powerful than ever, for it is the only sensuous experience that remains for him."[12] While we will quibble, in Key Seven, with the characterization that sexual diminishment is inevitable with aging, we agree that it's undeniable that touching needs to be a constant therapeutic tool for the health of both male and female senior citizens.

It certainly makes intuitive sense. After all, our skin is our largest body organ, "the oldest and most sensitive of our organs," contends Montagu, and "in the evolution of the senses the sense of touch was undoubtedly the first to come into being." He notes that a quarter-size piece of human skin contains three million cells, more than three hundred sweat glands, fifty nerve endings, and three feet of blood vessels. All these sensory receptors combine to instantly send information to the brain about heat, cold, pressure, pain, pleasure, and touch sensations.

"The communications we transmit through touch constitute the most powerful means of establishing human relationships, the foundation of experience," observes Montagu. "Where touching begins, there love and humanity also begin."[13] A sterling example of Montagu's observation comes from the life of Helen Keller. Blind and deaf since she was a toddler, Keller demonstrated later in life that she could effectively communicate with the outside world by using the touch of skin to compensate for her sensory deficiencies.

Children who grow up being touched only when they are disciplined by spanking or hitting often become adults who are warped in expressing sexuality. Some may grow up fearing physical contact and intimacy. Others may even get erotic or sexual gratification from having their skin abused, which may explain why sadism and masochism have become sexual outlets for certain segments of the population.

Finally, Montagu makes the point that nudism has its health benefits in freeing the skin to be caressed by the sun and air. "Clothes largely cut off the experience of pleasurable sensations from the skin, hence, the actual or symbolic shedding of clothes may represent attempts to enjoy experiences that had earlier been denied. Natural skin stimulation, the play of air, sun, and wind upon the body, can be very pleasurable....the growth of the nudist movement almost certainly reflects the desire for more freedom of communication through the skin."[14]

Reach Out and Touch Someone

Touch, using the practice of massage, releases powerful biochemicals that boost your immune system, enhance skin sensitivity, and nurture your ability to experience desire and arousal. Whether it's done in a therapeutic setting for nonsexual release or as sensual foreplay with your partner, massage provides one of the healthiest pathways to get in touch with your body and your feelings, while expanding your capacity for giving and receiving sexual energies and affectionate attention.

Massage is the most studied form of touch, and studies clearly show that it decreases stress hormones while raising the production of oxytocin, the "pleasure hormone." One of the more recent studies, published in the May 2008 issue of the *Journal of Alternative and Complementary Medicine*, administered blood tests before and after twenty-minute massages to a group of men ages nineteen to forty-five. A "significant increase" in oxytocin levels was detected in all the men after their massages, along with decreases in cortisol, the stress hormone.[15]

Since most standard massages performed by licensed massage therapists last for an hour or more, this limited yet revealing study examining the benefits of twenty minutes' worth of touching barely scratches the surface of therapeutic massage's potential for reducing anxiety and stress, and for releasing immune-boosting hormones such as oxytocin.

Some people come to Hippocrates never having had a massage in their life, which is truly sad given its therapeutic benefits to health. Giving massages, not just receiving them, also confers its own unique benefits to the giver's sexual health. A Hippocrates guest, Rebecca, fifty-eight, of Canton, Ohio, who describes herself as bisexual, outlines for us her work as a massage therapist and how healing touch communicates on multiple levels of awareness:

> I grew up in an extremely warm and loving family. The only sexual hang-up I had to overcome was the idea that oral sex was nasty, which my mother had impressed upon me. I grew up thinking that

massage was a natural part of lovemaking. I would rub anyone who would let me. It was only later in life that I discovered this wasn't natural for everyone. I didn't do massage to receive anything back. It was the tactile sensation that appealed to me. I love the sensation and smell of skin. It's all sensuous to me.

At the age of thirty-five, I became a professional massage therapist. But I couldn't let sensuality or sexuality come up while doing massages in a professional setting. So I had to learn how to control and channel the sexual energy that arises during massage sessions. But in my personal life, doing massages for my intimate partners, I can channel the sexual energy in a way that excites us both. Skin communicates beyond words. A lot of touching is important to creating a healthy sexual relationship. Massage should sometimes be just a sensual experience, rather than used as foreplay for releasing sexual tension. As a couple comes to understand the differences between sensuality and sexuality, they begin to generate the sort of foreplay between each other that can last a lifetime.

A bodywork therapist on our Hippocrates staff, Silvio, grew up in Brazil, a culture in which sexuality and nudity are not taboo subjects, but are treated as expressions of humankind's inherent sensual nature. Silvio may be more than sixty years old, yet the flame of libido still burns bright within him. It's a flame that he nourishes by dancing, which he calls "a way to feel my body and express sensuality through the joy of life."

Silvio offers our guests traditional Thai massage, whose roots can be traced back to what might seem to be a surprising source: monks. "People feel vitally charged from this massage technique," Silvio explains. "My work is not just to help them physically, but to help them to empower themselves. Monks in Thailand started this massage tradition long ago. This is also a spiritual tradition that holds the body to be sacred, and from that comes sensuality. It's the expression of God within us. Sensuality and sexuality are doors we can enter to the divine."

Are You Having a "Lust" Affair with a Vibrator?

Undoubtedly no one has studied the use of vibrators for sexual pleasuring among both women and men as much as Dr. Debby Herbenick, associate director of the Center for Sexual Health Promotion at Indiana University, Bloomington.

Her findings, presented in five separate coauthored studies published in medical journals, may surprise you.

About half of all women regularly use vibrators. Among Herbenick's sample of 2,056 women aged eighteen to sixty years, the prevalence of vibrator use was 52.5 percent, and this use was "associated with health-promoting behaviors and positive sexual function, and rarely associated with side effects." Nearly 30 percent of the women did report some genital symptoms, such as desensitization, from vibrator use.[16]

Around 44.8 percent of men sampled incorporate vibrator use into sexual activities during their lives. This was based on a survey of 1,047 men aged eighteen to sixty years in the United States. Such use occurred during both solo and partnered sexual interactions. Men who more commonly used vibrators "scored higher on four of the five domains of the International Index of Erectile Function (erectile function, intercourse satisfaction, orgasmic function, and sexual desire)."[17]

Male vibrator users often use the devices to accompany sexual intercourse. A survey discovered that 82 percent of men who had used a vibrator did so during sexual intercourse, which "supports the work of therapists and educators who often make recommendations for the incorporation of vibrators into partnered relationships."[18]

Women who have sex primarily with other women and use vibrators have higher sexual functioning scores than women who reported no vibrator use or vibrator use only during masturbation. These results were based on a survey of 2,192 women in Britain and the United States who had engaged in sexual activities only with women during the previous year.[19]

Another study revealed that about half of gay and bisexual men use vibrators, either solo or with a partner. Data was collected from 25,294 self-identified gay and bisexual men representing all fifty U.S. states. Three-fourths of the men had inserted the vibrators into their rectum during masturbation. Men reported that "vibrator use contributed to sexual arousal, orgasm and pleasure."[20]

A Kiss Isn't Just Pressing Lips Together

When you kiss someone, or someone kisses you, it can be like a comma, a question mark, or an exclamation point, the French actress Mistinguett once commented.

The first known written depictions of kissing appeared in Sanskrit around 1500 BC in India, followed centuries later by the *Kama Sutra*, a dating manual for bachelors, that identified seventeen different kisses and kissing techniques. Both ancient Greek and Roman pornographic murals portrayed kissing as an essential stage in the sexual act.

Why did this intimate exchange of saliva evolve into a symbol of love and bonding, and an invitation to express sexual behaviors? Anthropologists and evolutionary biologists offer several theories. Maybe kissing originated from our ancient forebears chewing food and passing it mouth to mouth to their babies, the way some species of animals do. Or maybe it's a form of social bonding that is instinctive.

Whatever the original motivation, most of us spend about two entire weeks out of an average life span engaged in kissing, according to Andrea Demirjian's book *Kissing: Everything You Ever Wanted to Know about One of Life's Sweetest Pleasures.*[21] But not all humans do it, or at least admit to it. Some tribal cultures in Asia, Africa, and South America regard the pressing of two pairs of lips together to be a disgusting or unhealthy practice.

At one time, kissing was considered a spiritual act in the Christian church. During the first few centuries of the church's existence, according to Michael Penn, author of *Kissing Christians: Ritual and Community in the Late Ancient Church*, Christians greeted each other, regardless of gender or age, with a "holy kiss," which they regarded as the passing of the Holy Spirit between two people.[22] Early Christians kissed during prayers, baptisms, and funerals and used just about any occasion as an opportunity to press lips together. Until the early sixteenth century, the holy kiss remained a ritual in the Catholic Mass, though outside that ritual, kissing had by then become formal, like a handshake.

63

The most notorious of all kisses, the tongue-probing French kiss, may not have originated with the French, but as with most anything that creative culture touches, the people of that region left their imprint on it. Using the tongue to explore another person's mouth, lips, or tongue was called cataglottis, from *cata* (meaning "down") and *glottis* (meaning "throat"). It's an act that has come to symbolize passion almost as much as sexual intercourse.

What no one realized, at least until twentieth-century medical science made the discovery, is that kissing sends chemical signals from one brain to another to stimulate sensations and moods and, more important, to assess the biological compatibility of a prospective sex partner and mate.

Our lips "are among the most densely populated with sensory neurons of any body region," reports *Scientific American Mind*. "When we kiss, these neurons, along with those in the tongue and mouth, rocket messages to the brain and body, setting off delightful sensations, intense emotions and physical reactions. Of the 12 or 13 cranial nerves that affect cerebral function, five are at work when we kiss, shuttling messages from our lips, tongue, cheeks and nose to a brain that snatches information about the temperature, taste, smell and movements of the entire affair."[23]

Kissing is a proven stress reducer, lowering cortisol levels in the bodies of both sexes. The act also produces oxytocin in males, which helps them to form feelings of attachment and devotion (women don't seem to need more oxytocin for that purpose). Other hormones and neurotransmitters released by kissing in both sexes are dopamine, essential to the processing of pleasure and emotion; serotonin, a mood and feeling enhancer; and adrenaline, which helps to dilate blood vessels and produce euphoria.

What lessons can we draw from these and other medical findings?

For one thing, the bigger your lips and tongue (collagen injections don't count), the more pleasure you can give and receive, if you practice.

Second, the more you make out, the more sensory hormones you stimulate, heightening overall foreplay pleasure, bonding with your partner, and intensifying the eventual sexual act.

Third, the more kissing you do with a committed partner, the more you strengthen each other's immune system. (Promiscuous deep kissing with strangers isn't recommended because the exchange of saliva, with its bacteria colonies, can pass on mononucleosis, that viral glandular fever sometimes known as the "kissing disease.")

Last, by inducing your partner to engage in prolonged and passionate kissing, you increase the chances of that person (especially if he is a male) remaining bonded to you. This is both a known psychological result and also a chemical consequence of the hormones released by kissing.

Train Your Brain's Love Chemical

Without the hormone oxytocin (Latin for "quick birth"), we wouldn't bond with other people or fall in love, according to research done at the National Institute of Mental Health.[24]

We release copious amounts of the hormone when we have orgasms, which helps to explain why sexual intimacy facilitates pair bonding. Mothers release it when breastfeeding, and a synthetic form of it, pitocin, is administered to some women to help promote contractions during childbirth.

Oxytocin has made an appearance in a commercially available form as a nasal spray sold over the Internet. At the Center for Neuroeconomics Studies in Claremont, California, volunteers who inhaled small doses of the oxytocin spray experienced reduced anxiety and shyness and became more generous and trusting.[25]

But nasal sprays are just a quick-fix shortcut. Natural activities release healthy amounts of oxytocin in us: making love, receiving massages, even petting an animal or holding a baby. Mind-body therapies such as yoga and breathing exercises also produce some of the same healthy effects.

Sex is a far more effective and healthier "medicine" than a synthetic nasal spray. It's a lot more fun and burns more calories, too!

Foreplay Should Last a Lifetime

Your mind is the first muscle to train in foreplay, so that it can use fantasy to enhance your experience of sexuality. Being able to fantasize with your partner, whether it's about other partners or other sexual situations, and talking about that during foreplay or sex are considered signals of good communication. Though sex hotlines are shallow forms of sexual communication, they obviously fill a need people have for such connection. (Needless to say, fantasy crosses a line when it becomes aggressive or violent.)

Here are three more foreplay rituals to try:

1. Take a warm bath, either alone or with a partner, using essential oils before intimacy. Certain essential oil scents expand sexual feelings: lavender, ylang-ylang, and vanilla are good examples.
2. Jump on a trampoline or do another form of aerobic exercise to get your lymphatic system moving. Preferably do this in the nude with your partner.
3. Try using feathers on your mate's body: just lightly touch the feather for ten minutes to heighten sensuality until both of you are ready to explode.

Seven Big Sexual Incompatibility Warning Signs

All couples experience a natural ebb and flow in their feelings of sexual connection to and desire for each other. Usually we can overlook any disconnect until time bridges the sex gap, or until we talk our way through the dry patch in intimacy. But if mutual disinterest or lopsided libidos persist, or if one partner becomes even more emotionally and physically withdrawn, and if months or years of lapsed desire pass, something is clearly wrong. It needs to be addressed or both partners run the risk of developing health and relationship impairments.

Here are seven of the most common warning signs of possible sexual incompatibility, according to a consensus view of sexologists:

1. The most obvious sign: your marriage has become sexless, which therapists often define as having sexual relations fewer

than ten times a year. If one or both partners undergo sex therapy and it doesn't help, then the incompatibility will probably be permanent, and you must learn to either "love it or leave it."

2. One partner wants to communicate about his or her bedroom desires as a prelude to expressing them, but the other partner can't or won't communicate with equal openness and honesty. Again, a sex therapist might be able to help.

3. One or both of you are rarely in the mood for sex. The reason could be a lack of real chemistry and attraction between you. Also see "Top Ten Libido Killers" on page 68 for other reasons that the mood is missing in action.

4. One of you grew up as a free spirit, uninhibited about sex, while the other partner was raised in a repressive home or was taught that sex is shameful. A sex therapist might be able to help the repressed partner to overcome guilty feelings or a poor body image, but this takes a strong commitment by both partners.

5. Psychological trauma or physical injury can dramatically alter a couple's sexual habits and feelings of compatibility. Both partners in such a situation could use therapy to heal and reconnect, or they could experiment with a broader range of sexual activities that might stimulate mutual satisfaction.

6. One of you is sexually dysfunctional, which could mean impotence in men or an inability to orgasm in women. These are not insurmountable problems, as this book documents. Sexual incompatibility resulting from these dysfunctions is more of a choice made by one or both partners than it is an inevitable consequence of the dysfunction.

7. One of you has sexual compulsions that cannot be controlled. The man may forego sex with his wife because he has an addictive compulsion to view pornography as he masturbates, rationalizing that he needs the excitement of sexual variety and graphic visual imagery. Or the woman may feel compelled

to have numerous sexual affairs outside of marriage — with or without her husband's knowledge — because she feels the need to constantly reaffirm her body image and her seductive appeal. Needless to say, these behaviors can put any relationship at risk if the partner cannot control his or her actions. Sex therapy is needed in these situations, or the incompatibility can become permanent.

Top Ten Libido Killers

1. **Stress.** How can you enjoy spontaneous intimacy and stay in the sexual moment if thoughts of deadlines, unpaid bills, or related worries obsessively haunt you? Even though sex and orgasms are proven stress relievers, if you can't summon the desire to perform, you won't get the relief you need.

2. **Depression.** A classic symptom of high- or low-level depression is loss of interest in sex. When you don't feel good about yourself or your life, mental and physical fatigue sets in, depleting your energy. That can't but help dampen your enthusiasm for and interest in pleasuring yourself or someone else. If the depression persists for weeks, it is important to seek medical or psychological assistance.

3. **Poor body image.** Low self-esteem can certainly undermine your libido. Few of us are always content with our bodies and how we look. Throughout life, we make adjustments with new exercise regimens, new hairstyles, new clothes and fashion. But if we are ashamed of our bodies, no amount of exterior change will mask the inner feeling of inadequacy. You may be able to hide your body from your partner for a while without consequences for the relationship, but unless you get right with yourself, poor body image can result in a vanishing libido.

4. **Excessive alcohol.** This should be an easy one to grasp. Whether you use recreational drugs or alcohol to excess, their

deadening effects will become obvious over time. Combine excessive usage with the slower recovery rates endemic to aging, and you have a recipe for a libido that is passed out drunk all the time.

5. Medication effects. Both prescription drugs and over-the-counter medications can undermine your appetite for sex. The worst offenders are tranquilizers and antidepressants such as Xanax, Prozac, and Paxil. These drugs can also short-circuit orgasms. Medications for hypertension, along with sedatives and opiates, can also have an impact on your normal levels of desire.

6. Oral contraceptives. Women who take the Pill stop more than their ovulation. Because this medication affects the ovaries, it affects the ovaries' hormone-producing ability. In response to the medication, women's bodies produce a protein called SHBG, according to Dr. Irwin Goldstein, coeditor of *Women's Sexual Function and Dysfunction*. This protein binds itself to sex hormones. The result can be a diminished sex drive.[26]

7. Medical conditions. High cholesterol, diabetes, thyroid disorders, and autoimmune disorders are the primary culprits. Few people feel very sexy when they're distracted by pain or the symptoms of medical conditions.

8. Childbirth and mothering. Genital sensitivity may be reduced after giving birth. Not only that, but lower estrogen levels in lactating women can dry out the vaginal opening and contribute to a lower sex drive. Medical authorities also point out that breastfeeding increases production of the hormone prolactin, another libido-lowering agent.

9. Bedroom boredom. You can't just do the same thing over and over again and expect to keep yourself or your partner interested. It's not just a cliché to say that variety is the spice of life. Variety truly is the bedroom spice that is essential to a stimulated and healthy libido. If your imagination isn't up to

the task of breaking the boredom spell, consult other sections and resources in this book for some provocative ideas.

10. **A toxic diet.** There are particular foods that enhance your libido and your sexual performance, and other foods that are toxic to the libido. Fast food, junk food, processed food — all the usual suspects combine to clog your arteries and toxify your libido. The cleaner your food, the healthier your libido. People who have been living a healthy lifestyle for long periods of time rarely complain about a loss of libido.

What's Your Sexual Intercourse Time?

Studies have been done throughout the world to measure the average amount of time heterosexual couples engage in sexual intercourse, and it's the women who have been holding the stopwatches.

Dutch researchers recruited five hundred couples from five countries — Britain, the Netherlands, Spain, Turkey, and the United States — and armed the female partners with stopwatches to time each bout of intercourse over a four-week period. Special attention was paid to whether the couples used condoms and whether the men were circumcised.

The results were published in the July 2005 issue of the *Journal of Sexual Medicine* and revealed the following titillating facts:

- The average duration of sexual intercourse, defined as the time between the start of penetration and ejaculation, was 5.4 minutes for all the couples.
- The median duration wasn't affected by condom use or by whether the man was circumcised.
- Couples in Turkey devoted the shortest average amount of time, 3.7 minutes, to intercourse among the five countries.
- When average times were broken down based on age, 6.5 minutes was the average time for the eighteen- to thirty-year-olds, compared to 4.3 minutes on average for those couples older than fifty-one.[27]

So, given these study results, what would you guess most sex therapists would recommend as the optimal or "normal" intercourse duration?

That question motivated some Penn State University researchers to survey members of the Society for Sex Therapy and Research in the United States and Canada. Here's the consensus opinion of these sex therapists about what's normal or abnormal, as published in the May 2008 issue of the *Journal of Sexual Medicine*:

- Without including foreplay, an "adequate" period for intercourse was said to be three to seven minutes in duration.
- An intercourse period considered "too short" was one to two minutes, while "too long" was defined as any sexual union lasting more than ten minutes.[28]

It's hard to imagine why sex therapists would offer an opinion that ten minutes or more of sexual pleasure is "too long" and thus not normal or natural. Apparently, they must think that sexual marathons are a symptom of addictive behavior. Either that, or their own sex lives leave a lot to be desired.

Your Nose Is a Sex Organ

Most people overlook or underestimate the powerful role that our sense of smell plays in the wonderful dance of life that is romance and the expression of sexuality.

At the most basic level, chemical reaction, smells are just volatile molecules that provide clues about the identity of what emitted them. But we humans instinctively assign values to these smells, recoiling from the smell of excrement, for instance, while being attracted to the scent of flowers.

Studies have shown that males use their sense of smell to know instinctively when females are ready to conceive, and women tend to be most attracted to smells associated with men who are genetically compatible with them. When we feel the "sexual chemistry" of attraction to another person, we are picking up a scent-based recognition of potential biological compatibility.

Did You Know?

Soy Can Warp the Female Sex Drive

Eating soy can depress sexual desire in some women, while in others soy can drive their sexuality to the Indianapolis 500 raceway.

First, the depressing news. Though you may not be directly related to a rat, the effects of soy supplements on female rats are similar to the effects observed in some human females.

Isoflavones, a key compound in soy, are estrogen-like molecules that have been shown in laboratory experiments at Emory University in Atlanta to interfere with normal estrogen function in rats. Sexual behaviors were reduced by up to 70 percent in female rats given the commercially available doses of soy supplements that many women take.[29]

Since women usually take soy supplements to counteract the symptoms of menopause, it's difficult for them to know if reductions in their sex drive are due to the soy or to menopause. Sometimes, probably, it's a combination of both.

But soy can also be a contributing factor to a condition in women called persistent sexual arousal syndrome. A 2005 article in the *Journal of Sexual Medicine* described a forty-four-year-old woman who began adding large amounts of soy to her diet. One month later, she felt such intense sexual cravings that she was masturbating to orgasm up to fifteen times a day. Once she discontinued these phytoestrogens in her diet, her sexuality returned to normal.[30]

Psychologist Rachel Herz, author of *The Scent of Desire*, has made the point that smells we usually think are attractive generally come from people who are most genetically compatible with us. It has even been shown by researchers in Sweden that homosexual men and many heterosexual women have a scent-based ability to "sniff out" the sexual orientation of people they have just met.[31]

Natural body odor is also a by-product of our dietary choices. Anecdotal accounts and our experience with guests at the Hippocrates Health Institute support the idea that vegans possess a cleaner natural smell than do meat and dairy product consumers, perhaps because their immune systems are stronger. The same anecdotal evidence has been true for the flavor of body fluids — among vegans, women's vaginal secretions and men's semen taste less bitter and more honey-like than secretions from meat and dairy eaters.

Why are some aromas sexually stimulating? That's a mystery being explored by research led by Dr. Alan Hirsch, author of *Scentsational Sex*, at the Smell and Taste Treatment and Research Foundation in Chicago, which has shown that certain aromas, such as cinnamon, affect the biochemistry of humans in a way that stimulates desire. Certain combinations of odors create the strongest effects on human sexual arousal; two of the most powerful combinations are lavender and pumpkin, and licorice and pumpkin.

Thirty-one men aged eighteen to sixty-four years were recruited for the experiment that Dr. Hirsch and his colleague, Dr. Jason Gruss, conducted to determine which of thirty odors most increases blood flow to the penis. Each man was hooked up to a plethysmograph (a device that measures penile blood flow) and then breathed into a mask through which odors were randomly supplied. The mixed odor of lavender and pumpkin had the greatest effect, increasing arousal and blood flow by 40 percent on average. The aroma with the least impact on sexual arousal was cranberry, with just 2 percent increased arousal.[32]

Aromas associated with certain essential oils have been clinically proven to be human mood enhancers, which might be useful during foreplay to stimulate sexual desire and to enhance sexual performance. Here are two study examples:

- A January 2008 study published in the *International Journal of Neuroscience* reported that the aroma of peppermint essential oil "significantly increased calmness" in human test subjects. Peppermint also enhanced memory. One hundred forty-three volunteers had their mood, memory, and alertness tested before and after inhalation of peppermint and ylang-ylang aromas. Whereas peppermint enhanced both memory and alertness and increased calmness, ylang-ylang decreased both memory and alertness.[33]

- In a January 2003 study published in the *International Journal of Neuroscience*, the essential oils lavender and rosemary were tested on 143 volunteers. Researchers found both aromas stimulated a mood of contentment in most of the test subjects. Lavender decreased memory and impaired reaction times in the test subjects, but had a calming effect on their mood and elevated their levels of contentment. Rosemary produced a "significant enhancement of performance for overall quality of memory," according to the researchers, but also benefitted mood and contentment.[34]

A next step in this research field might be to measure the effects of these essential oils on stimulating sexual desire. In the Ayurvedic medicine tradition of India, cardamom, champa, ginger, and vanilla are among the essential oils long considered to be aphrodisiacs.

There is a "stealth" technology at work today that confounds our ability to use the powers of smell to sense biological and sexual compatibility — it's the thousands of synthetic chemical aromas that are added to the personal care products, colognes, perfumes, and cosmetics that most people use every day. Could this be a factor in the skyrocketing rates of divorce? Do these synthetic scents hide natural body odors that normally provide evidence of incompatibility? More research is needed.

High Female Sex Drive Can Produce Bisexuality

Women with higher than average sex drives are more likely to be bisexual than men with high sex drives, and they have a greater tendency toward bisexuality than women with "normal" to low libidos.

A series of studies published in the journals *Archives of Sexual Behavior* (2007), *Psychological Science* (2006), and elsewhere reached this conclusion after assessing survey results from 3,645 U.S. men and women of all self-identified sexual orientations. These findings were subsequently replicated in large international surveys that spanned many different countries, age groups, and cultural traditions.[35]

Why would a high sex drive in women be associated with an increased sexual attraction to both men and women? Theories abound. Here are two from Richard Lippa, a psychologist at California State University, Fullerton, who authored the articles:

- "Women tend to be more flexible and variable in their same-sex and other-sex attractions than men," perhaps because "the neural and hormonal processes that underlie the development of sexual orientation differ for men and women."
- An additional reason could be that "male sexual orientation may result, in part, from gender socialization that is more rigid and rigorous for boys than for girls and from socialization zealots who disapprove more strongly of feminine behaviors in boys and men than they do of masculine behaviors in girls and women. Such socialization pressures could lead heterosexual men to suppress same-sex attractions more than heterosexual women do."[36]

Heal Sexual Dysfunctions with Hypnosis

Hundreds of controlled medical studies have documented that hypnotic sessions conducted by trained hypnotherapists, and sometimes self-hypnosis performed by people on their own, can help to heal maladies and disorders ranging from irritable bowel syndrome, nausea, and autoimmune dysfunction to warts and weight problems.

Add to this list sexual dysfunctions such as frigidity, an inability to climax in women, and erectile problems in men. If there is a psychological cause for the dysfunction, or if a blockage exists in the unconscious mind that impedes healing, then hypnosis may be a useful tool for you to try.

A British hypnotherapist, Dr. Shaun Brookhouse, director of training and research at the Washington School of Clinical and Advanced Hypnosis, provides a case example of how hypnosis relieved a profound state of sexual dysfunction in a woman he calls Janet. She had lost all sexual feelings for her partner after many years of being together. She seemed too young to be going through menopause, so her physician suggested that hypnotherapy might get to the root of why she had lost sexual desire.

Dr. Brookhouse did a progressive relaxation program in which he gave her suggestions that relaxed each part of her body. Though she had never been hypnotized before, the first session of forty-five minutes went well and a second session was scheduled. After the first session, though she had no change in feelings toward her partner, she was able to sleep more easily. This was a clue for Dr. Brookhouse that Janet's sexual dysfunction was rooted in her past and not in the present.

He did regressive hypnosis in which he took her back into her memory, starting at the age of thirty-five. As he counted down, he asked her to indicate whether any sexual trauma had occurred at that age by raising an index finger. At the age of twenty-one, her index finger stood up and she began to cry. At that age she had been sexually assaulted in a college dormitory room.

A third hypnotic session provided more details of the assault. Dr. Brookhouse discovered that the room in which she was assaulted had light green walls. He asked her to describe her bedroom at home that she shared with her partner. "It is light blue," said Janet, then she stopped herself. "No," she corrected, "my partner just repainted it light green." It took only a few more questions for Dr. Brookhouse to put everything together. Janet's sexual dysfunction began shortly after the repainting of her bedroom to a color that closely matched the walls where her assault had occurred years earlier. The lack of desire for her partner had been triggered by the psychological cue of his repainting of the bedroom.

"Not all cases of psychological sexual dysfunction are so easy to resolve," comments Dr. Brookhouse on his webpage, www.hypno-nlp .com. "Not all sexual dysfunction is psychological. If you suffer from sexual dysfunction, ask for your medical practitioner's opinion as to its cause. If it is psychological, be sure that you consult a properly qualified therapist. When looking for a therapist to assist you with sexual dysfunc- tion, please ensure that the therapist treats the situation with a great deal of kindness and compassion."[37]

To learn more about the use of hypnosis in finding sexual fulfillment, you might read the book *Hypnosex: Sexual Joy through Self-Hypnosis*, by Daniel L. Araoz and Robert Bleck, which can be found on Amazon.com.[38]

EXERCISE: MAKE MASSAGE YOUR FOREPLAY RITUAL

You and your partner can sensually massage each other's bodies and stimulate your libidos in a variety of ways to help keep your relation- ship intimate and vital. For best results, turn this into a regular ritual as a prelude to sexual intimacy.

Dozens of how-to books and DVDs can teach you the basics of massage techniques, so we won't repeat any of that advice or instruc- tion here. It's important, however, to distinguish between therapeu- tic massage and sensual massage. Therapeutic massage isn't intended to inspire sexual activity, whereas sensual massage can, though not necessarily must, lead to sexual activity.

Start by renting or buying an instructional DVD describing how to perform a sensual massage. Practice the techniques. Then prepare yourselves for the experience. Ambience and a proper setting are keys to creating and enhancing mood.

Pick a quiet room and turn down the lights, or do the massage by candlelight. Play soft, tranquil mood music, or music that you know heightens your partner's senses. Make certain the phones are turned off and you won't be interrupted by relatives or friends. Be sure to be patient and loving, and devote sufficient time for the massage to produce maximum relaxation and heightened sensitivity.

Don't directly stimulate the genitals. Foreplay is about teasing and being suggestive. Your goal is to increase sexual tension until, when you finally have sexual release, it's a memorable experience. Variations can include blindfolding your partner, or using a scarf or feather to perform the massage before you use your hands.

Experiment with awakening your partner's senses, make it a sacred ritual in your lives, and you will create an entirely new level of affection, bonding, and sexual intimacy.

Protect Your Sexuality

An orgasm a day keeps the doctor away.

— Actress Mae West (1893–1980)

Toxins Short-Circuit Sexuality

We are all by nature sexual beings, but this natural gift is subject to a host of outside influences that can sabotage our sexual functioning, and even our sexual orientation. There is no doubt in our minds that infertility and impotence happen in great part because of chemicals and radioactivity in our environment.

We all carry a synthetic chemical body burden that we have absorbed from contact with foods, municipal water supplies, medicines, cosmetics, personal care products, and other consumer items. For each of us, that means seven hundred or more of these chemicals have taken up residence in our body fat and body organs at any one time, according to estimates from the U.S. Centers for Disease Control and Prevention, which has conducted widespread blood testing on thousands of people over the past decade.[1]

The toxic effects of these chemicals and our body burdens' imposi-
tions on sexuality and sexual health are finally being recognized and documented. The following information is what every one of us needs to be
aware of if we intend to be sexually active until the end of our lives.

Some of the synthetic chemicals that we absorb are hormone disrupters, which means they play havoc with our sex glands. More than a decade
ago, researchers at Case Western Reserve University in Cleveland acci-
dentally discovered that bisphenol A (BPA), a chemical used in the plastic
coatings of food containers and baby bottles, can cause reproductive and
sex abnormalities in rodents.[2]

An entire class of petroleum by-products called phthalates (pronounced "thallets"), used in plastics and cosmetics, has been linked to
gender-bender effects in humans, even at very low doses and exposure
levels. In 2005, for example, the scientific journal *Environmental Health
Perspectives* contained a study from the University of Rochester showing
that 134 boys with sex abnormalities such as tiny testicles and tiny penises
had been exposed in the womb to higher-than-normal levels of phthalates
absorbed by their mothers.[3] Another study, in 2003 at the Harvard School
of Public Health, documented phthalate levels in 168 males at a fertility
clinic, finding that men with the highest levels were five times more likely
than those with low levels to have low sperm counts that undermined
their ability to father children.[4]

British newspapers reported in 2005 that clinics in London had more
than doubled their numbers of male patients seeking breast reduction surgery. Female hormones from contraceptive pills flushed into the sewer
system and then recycled into London's drinking water were one possible
cause. Another cause may have been rising levels of estrogen-mimicking
chemicals these men were exposed to in their foods and personal care
products.[5] At least fifty chemicals in common usage throughout the world
have been documented to be hormone disruptive.

As detailed in Randall Fitzgerald's 2007 book *The Hundred-Year
Lie: How to Protect Yourself from the Chemicals That Are Destroying Your
Health*, hormone-disruptive effects first showed up in wildlife populations

several decades ago. In the 1990s, hermaphroditic fish appeared in the Great Lakes, and, more recently, they turned up in large numbers off the coast of California and in the Potomac River near Washington, D.C. Biologists concluded these gender-bender effects were the result of contact with estrogen-mimicking chemicals being pumped into those bodies of water.[6] A similar phenomenon of hermaphroditic wildlife has been occurring throughout Europe.

Research done in 2005 by biologists at Washington State University revealed an even more alarming discovery. Rats exposed to a hormone-disruptive insecticide and fungicide passed the exposure effects to their offspring by a change in their DNA code. Ninety percent of male offspring were born with low sperm counts or abnormal sperm production, or were completely infertile. This infertility was then passed down to second-, third-, and fourth-generation males via DNA alteration.[7]

We live in a microscopic cesspool in which manmade chemistry is replacing healthy microorganisms. When a person is weakened at any level by chemical exposure, sexual vitality seems to be the first bodily function to suffer.

Young men in their thirties come in to see us with erectile dysfunction, and young women in their thirties with early menopause. There is a trend of asexuality among people in their twenties, and the vast majority may be suffering from exposure to environmental toxins that erase sexual desire. The impact of hormone-disrupting chemicals cannot be overlooked.

The penis and clitoris are like thermometers measuring health threats. Penis sizes are decreasing, and endocrine disrupters are affecting the anal-genital distance standards of normality. In just a couple of generations, we've dropped five years in the average age of menarche. Younger bodies are becoming more sexual without comparable emotional development.

Toxins affect both the ability to orgasm and the intensity of orgasm. White blood cells are a key — they are the birthplace of eggs and sperm — and we've seen white blood cell counts getting lower over the past few decades, according to results from blood testing we have conducted at Hippocrates.

Pharmaceutical drugs play a role, too. More than half the people in this country are on medications. These often undermine sexual desire and performance. The most common side effect of many pharmaceuticals is a reduction of sexual potency and desire. Some medical studies estimate that prescription drugs account for at least 25 percent of all sexual problems in men and women, affecting both sexual desire and sexual functioning. Classes of drugs most often associated with loss of sexual desire and the creation of sexual dysfunctions are antidepressants, sedatives, anxiolytics, and antihypertensive medications.

Endocrine-disrupting chemicals that make your hormones go haywire appear in everyday products, too, especially cosmetics and personal care products. Dr. Samuel Epstein's book *Toxic Beauty: How Cosmetics and Personal-Care Products Endanger Your Health* documents how hundreds of products most people take for granted and use every day contain chemical threats to sexuality and sexual health. Among the more common hormone disrupters are, again, phthalates.

Dr. Epstein cites medical evidence "that men with high levels of phthalates in their urine had reduced sperm counts, low sperm motility, and more deformed sperm. A subsequent pilot study reported genital abnormalities in male babies whose mothers were found to have high levels of four phthalate by-products."

About thirty hormone-disruptive chemicals are found in products sold as nonorganic. Here is a partial list, based on Dr. Epstein's research, of product categories commonly containing hormone disrupters:

- perfumes
- body lotions
- sunscreens
- deodorant
- shampoo
- lipstick
- nail polish

- hairspray
- cologne
- aftershave[8]

"Use It or Lose It" Isn't Just a Cliché

Imagine two people playing ball. If one individual leaves the game, you can no longer play with the same intensity. The same rule applies to sexual activity. If you are only sexually active alone, over time you lose the ability to play with a partner. If you aren't even sexually active by yourself, you lose the ability to be sexual at all. The longer you abstain from sex, the lower your hormone and sperm or egg production. You ultimately lose your sexual chemistry potential, and that affects your health.

Massachusetts Male Aging Study senior researcher Dr. Irwin Goldstein concludes from his work that lifestyle-related diseases, rather than aging, constitute the most preventable reason for impotence in men. His study found that male testosterone levels are raised by sexual intercourse, and that those men who don't regularly engage in sexual activity experienced dramatic drops in testosterone levels as the years passed.[9] This is another reason to use it or lose it.

One of the clearest pieces of medical evidence yet that men who don't frequently use their sexual equipment lose their ability to do so comes from a Finnish study published in the *American Journal of Medicine* in July 2008. Nearly one thousand Finnish men aged fifty-five to seventy-five years were studied over a five-year period and evaluated for their sexual frequency and subsequent risk of erectile dysfunction. The impotence rate was seventy-nine per one thousand among men who had sex less than once a week, compared to thirty-two per thousand in men having weekly sexual activity, and just sixteen per thousand among men having sex at least three times a week.

The six researchers at a Finnish hospital who conducted the study conclude, "Regular intercourse protects against the development of erectile dysfunction among men aged 55 to 75 years. This may have an impact on general health and quality of life; therefore, doctors should support patients' sexual activity."[10]

Three Types of Sexual Dysfunction and Their Symptoms

Both men and women can experience three types of sexual dysfunctions: disorders of desire, disorders of arousal, and disorders of orgasm, according to the three female health practitioners who coauthored *The New Harvard Guide to Women's Health*:

1. **Disorders of desire.** These are typified by a lack of libido or interest in sex. Women with low libidos, a condition called hypoactive sexual desire disorder, rarely if ever have sexual fantasies or show an interest in sex. Usually this disorder is accompanied by disorders of arousal and orgasm. Men more often complain about a loss of desire than do women, according to the authors. A person's sex drive can be diminished by physical health issues, a loss of attraction to one's spouse, lifestyle changes, and mood disorders such as depression. Hormone changes can also play a role. Some people even develop phobias around sex in which they are repulsed by the idea of genital contact with another person.

2. **Disorders of arousal.** These include impotence in men and vaginal dryness and involuntary vaginal muscle contraction in women. Arousal problems can occur for many reasons. Anxiety about sexual performance can afflict both men and women. Attempting intercourse without adequate foreplay can exacerbate feelings of anxiety, as can concerns about pregnancy and sexually transmitted diseases. For women nearing or past menopause, hormonal deficiencies can impede arousal and vaginal lubrication. Depression, stress, and unexpressed anger toward a partner also contribute to problems with arousal.

Did You Know?

Why the G-Spot Remains Controversial

It was in 1950 that a German gynecologist, Ernst Grafenberg, published a paper in an obscure medical journal proposing that the anterior wall of a woman's vagina harbors a highly erogenous zone capable of inducing an orgasm similar to, but potentially more powerful than, a clitoral orgasm.[11]

The G-spot, as it became known, was later localized during autopsies of cadavers as being at the urethral sphincter muscle area in the vagina. During the 1970s, Professor Beverly Whipple, then of the College of Nursing at Rutgers University, did even more extensive research into the G-spot while training women to improve their pelvic muscle control.

Professor Whipple examined more than four hundred women and identified the G-spot about one-third of the way up inside the vagina, making it a sort of female prostate gland. Pressure on the underlying tissue causes it to swell and triggers orgasm in some but not all women.[12]

Because not all women can have their G-spot area activated, and perhaps because only a few sexual intercourse positions seem to trigger its sensitivity by pressure, many physicians have doubted the G-spot's very existence. Doubts also arose from a failure to identify nerve endings in that area corresponding to nerve endings in the clitoris. A survey of studies published in a 2001 issue of the *American Journal of Obstetrics & Gynecology* concludes that the elusive G-spot is "a sort of gynecologic UFO: much sought for, much discussed, but unverified by objective means."[13]

The answer to this debate must be provided on an individual basis by those women who have found their G-spot and use it to experience the deep, full-body orgasmic contractions that it affords.

3. Disorders of orgasm. These include difficulty in achieving orgasm in women and premature ejaculation in men. Unrealistic expectations about romance and the sexual act can cause some women difficulty in experiencing orgasms. An inability to relax or release distrust, fear, or anxiety can short-circuit

an orgasmic response to sexual stimulation. An estimated 40 percent of women must have direct clitoral stimulation to achieve orgasm, which means they require more foreplay to raise their excitement level. About 8 percent of women still cannot climax with direct clitoral stimulation, due to either physical or psychological factors. One treatment for orgasmic dysfunction is the practice of Kegel exercises (see Key Five) to develop vaginal muscles that facilitate orgasmic release.[14]

Will Sleeping Apart Affect Desire?

Maybe he snores so loudly that the neighborhood dogs howl and there's no way for you to get a good night's sleep. Or perhaps she's the culprit, and as you're falling asleep, she reflexively jerks her arm or her leg and smacks you in the head or groin as if she were practicing for the world karate championships. This person loves you and you love them back, but you can't sleep with them every night because you'll suffer at work the entire next day.

Sleep deprivation can take many forms and may result from stress, conflicting schedules, and a dozen other reasons. The consequences of sleeping with someone who disturbs your sleep pattern over an extended period can be disastrous to the relationship, most particularly to the sexual connection between you and your partner.

More couples than ever are choosing to sleep apart to protect their relationship and even their sanity. Surveys conducted by the National Sleep Foundation confirm this trend. A 2001 survey of 1,004 married couples discovered that 12 percent slept alone most of the time; by 2005, a similar poll by the same group found the numbers had nearly doubled, to 23 percent of respondents reporting separate sleeping arrangements.[15] The numbers were even higher in Britain, whose national Sleep Council documented that one in four couples regularly seek a good night's sleep by choosing to be alone in separate rooms most nights.[16]

What does sleeping apart with regularity do to a couple's sexuality? Does it necessarily result in trouble for the sexual connection they share and, ultimately, for the future of the relationship? Or can sleeping apart actually intensify desire and make the relationship more passionate than ever before?

Your answer to these questions may depend mostly on the strength of the bond you and your partner share outside of the bedroom. Minnesota marriage counselor Willard Harley Jr., author of *Love Busters: Overcoming the Habits That Destroy Romantic Love*, contends that sleeping together is an important aspect of feeling integrated with your partner.[17] Sleeping apart can be a symptom of a deeper disturbance in the relationship that can find expression in both partners seeking more excuses for time away from each other.

But sleeping apart periodically can also be a healthy sign of a mutual independence that might actually strengthen the relationship and make sex more exciting. When you're rested and not worrying about stress caused by a lack of quality sleep time, you may appreciate your partner more. That could inspire you to create "dates" for intimate encounters in which the goal is simply to enjoy each other sexually without feeling that it is an obligation or a routine. Much as happens when one partner goes away on a business trip, being apart in separate beds can stoke the imagination and inflame the libido as you look forward to being intimate with the person you desire and love.

Do You or Your Partner Have "Sexsomnia"?

At least eleven different sex-related sleep disorders have been identified over the past decade, such as conditions labeled "sexsomnia" or "sleep-sex" that cause otherwise psychologically healthy people to initiate sex with themselves or others while asleep, much as if they were sleepwalking.

As bizarre as it might sound that someone could have sleep sex all the way to orgasm and not remember anything about the encounter, this condition isn't as rare as you might think. It also has legal ramifications, since the sexual relations might be nonconsensual. According to a research report in the May 2007 issue of the journal *Behavior Research Methods*, "Sexsomnia may be quite common but often goes unreported because of shame and embarrassment."[18]

Three Canadian sleep researchers did a survey of 219 persons who had reported experiencing sexsomnia incidents. Their median age was thirty, and one-third of them were women. "The respondents typically reported multiple sexsomnia episodes, in most cases precipitated by body contact, stress and fatigue," the researchers wrote in the December 2007 issue of *Social Psychiatry & Psychiatric Epidemiology*. "Relatively small numbers of respondents reported involvement of the legal authorities (8.6% of males and 3% of females) and participation of minors in their sexsomnia (6% of total sample)."[19]

Further research by the Minnesota Regional Sleep Disorders Center, published in the June 2007 issue of the journal *Sleep*, identified the full range of sleep-related sexual behaviors for both men and women, including masturbation, erections and vaginal lubrication, fondling, intercourse with climax, and even sexual assault and rape, all with resultant amnesia about the experience.[20]

"Bizarre and inappropriate behavior during sleep does not necessarily reflect a daytime psychological problem," says psychiatrist Carlos Schenck, author of *Sleep: A Groundbreaking Guide to the Mysteries, the Problems, and the Solutions*.[21] But the longer a person who has a sex-related sleep disorder goes without seeking help, the greater the prospect that this condition might lead to serious secondary psychological problems, even serious legal problems if minors or sexual assaults are involved. Schenck believes that sexsomnia disorders can be effectively treated with certain types of medication.

Negative Thoughts or Feelings Sabotage Orgasms

Whether you're male or female, being unable to experience orgasmic release during sexual activity can produce a sense of frustration, inadequacy, helplessness, and even depression. Those feelings can further suppress your ability to have an orgasm because negativity feeds upon itself, and that vicious cycle can be difficult to break.

If you have an underlying fear of intimacy that you haven't recognized or dealt with, you may actually dread the vulnerability that comes from sharing an orgasm with someone. This psychological aversion to orgasm could also be produced by prior sexual abuse, poor body image, or performance anxiety.

If your parents indoctrinated you with negative messages about sex and expressing your sexuality while you were growing up, your inhibited physical responses to stimulation could be a direct consequence. Guilt is one of those negative emotions that skewer healthy appreciation and expression of physical pleasures.

Maybe you're in denial about relationship issues you have with your partner or spouse. These unexpressed feelings, no matter how well you think you have buried them, can surge to the surface during intimate moments and short-circuit your orgasmic electrical system.

If any of these negative thought or feeling patterns seem to describe you and the sexual challenges you face, you may want to find a professional sex therapist in your area by consulting the American Association of Sexuality Educators, Counselors and Therapists' website at www.aasect.org.

Ten Reasons Orgasms Are Good for You

1. You will strengthen your immune system. Orgasms release hormones beneficial to immunity. DHEA (dehydroepiandrosterone), for instance, bolsters the immune system against colds and the flu and helps to maintain and repair body tissues. A study done at the Wilkes University Department of Psychology and published in *Psychological Reports* in June 2004 surveyed 112 college students on the frequency of their sexual encounters. Saliva samples were collected to test for the presence of immunoglobulin A (IgA), an antibody that protects against colds and infections. Those students reporting the greatest frequency of sexual activity, defined as two or

more times a week, showed "significantly higher" levels of IgA than those students who were less sexually active.[22]

2. You will reduce stress. You probably know this to be true from firsthand experience. Nothing quite as quickly and dramatically washes away the tensions of the day as the release that comes from lovemaking. You certainly rest better afterward.

3. You will relieve depression. The hormones released during lovemaking and orgasms elevate a person's mood sufficiently to dispel most symptoms of depression. If, however, the depression is severe or long-term, then it can prevent the intimacy necessary to produce an orgasm.

4. You will strengthen your body. Sexual intercourse requires a sequence of muscle contractions and movements for both men and women that provides a good source of exercise. Doing Kegel exercises, too, before and during sex can intensify orgasms and help to improve problems with incontinence and erectile dysfunction.

5. You will sleep better. Both men and women experience a drop in blood pressure after orgasm, though it occurs much faster in men. This drop, combined with the release of endorphins, is a great tranquilizer for people who have trouble falling asleep.

6. You will improve your sense of smell. Science has shown us the role that pheromones play in attraction and sexual chemistry. But did you know that new neurons develop in your brain's smell center in response to the release of prolactin, one of orgasm's hormones?

7. You will reduce your risk of heart attack. Numerous medical studies have found that having sex at least three times a week significantly lowers the risk of heart disease or a stroke. The combination of orgasm hormones and increased blood flow helps to keep the heart healthy.

8. You will lose weight. You've probably heard that you lose one pound of fat for every additional 3,500 calories that you burn. By most estimates, a half hour of sexual intercourse burns

about 150 calories, and even more if you're particularly vigorous in your lovemaking. So having sex three times a week may take off that pound of weight in just a couple of months.

9. You will relieve pain. When orgasms release oxytocin into your body, endorphins are secreted, and these natural opiates exercise an analgesic effect that is beneficial to reducing pain associated with arthritis, headaches, and other ailments.

10. You will live longer. As you will discover in Key Seven of this book, medical studies have accumulated impressive evidence that orgasm frequency is related to longevity. On average, people who have two or more orgasms a week have half the death rate of similarly aged people who experience orgasms only once a month.

Infamous Sex Myth

Paralyzed People Cannot Experience Orgasms

Stimulation of parts of the human body other than the genitals can produce orgasms.

That finding comes from research with a group of women who experienced spinal injuries and paralysis as a result of gunshot wounds. Professor Beverly Whipple, then at the College of Nursing at Rutgers University, found that some women can climax by using imagery in their minds alone. Others could experience orgasmic sensations when hypersensitive skin near the site of their injury was stimulated in just the right way.

One woman, who had been told by her physicians she would never have another orgasm because she had no feeling below the level of her breasts, experienced six orgasms during three twelve-minute sessions of genital and nongenital stimulation initiated by Professor Whipple in her laboratory.[23]

While this area of research is new and much more about the mysteries of orgasm remains to be uncovered, it offers hope for renewed sexual functioning for those who have been paralyzed, and it gives the rest of us reassurance that our entire mind-body connection can be an orgasmic trigger.

Did You Know?

An Orgasmic Chemical Produces Pleasure

In women, sexual stimulation and arousal release oxytocin, and a much higher level is released when orgasm occurs. For men, only orgasm and ejaculation of seminal fluid release oxytocin. That sex difference gives us a glimpse into why women usually desire more foreplay than men.

What makes this chemical special is that it stimulates the emotional centers of the brain in both men and women. That stimulation produces comforting feelings, relaxation, and a sense of being bonded to each other.

This chemical is a natural antistress neurotransmitter and helps us to cope with the stress that we feel in our everyday lives. Studies have found low levels of oxytocin in people experiencing anxiety disorders and anorexia nervosa.

How Food Can Safeguard Sexual Desire

If you ever saw the movie *The Taming of the Shrew*, with Elizabeth Taylor and Richard Burton, which is set in Elizabethan Britain, you may recall the dining scene in which the two main characters engage in a bawdy bite-for-bite buildup of erotic desire that results in passionate sex. Food has traditionally been connected to sexual arousal in both art and reality throughout recorded human history, yet what is much less known or acknowledged is the link that exists among high-fat foods, cardiovascular disease, and impotence. Most of the factors that predispose people to strokes and heart attacks — a high-fat diet, obesity, lack of exercise, high blood pressure — also work against the maintenance of sexual functioning.

Shari Lieberman, PhD, a New York nutrition scientist and physiologist, brings the food and sex link into sharp focus: "Sexual function depends on the cardiovascular system, the heart and blood vessels, and the nervous system — the body's electrical wiring. Good food choices can keep these sexually crucial systems functioning at their best, but bad ones can poison them."[24]

Four Food Types That Poison Sex

Consuming the following "food" types over time will have a cumulative impact on your body that can produce impotence in men and less genital sensitivity in women.

1. All fatty meats. Whether it's bacon or sausage or beef, the saturated fats and cholesterol in fatty meat will narrow the arteries in your penis or vaginal area faster than anything else, because these arteries are some of the smallest in your body and collect plaque very quickly. Sometimes the effects of these fats on sexual performance can be observed and felt immediately after consuming a single high-fat meal. Symptoms include taking longer to be aroused, difficulty in maintaining arousal, and trouble achieving orgasm.

2. All dairy products. The saturated fats in most cheeses and varieties of milk rival the fatty meats in narrowing your arteries. Probably a true nightmare for your sex life is a meal such as a bacon cheeseburger with French fries, washed down by a milkshake. If you've ever had such a meal, can you remember having had sex in the hours following it? Odds are it wasn't a memorable experience, or if it was memorable, then for the wrong reasons.

3. All processed baked goods. Don't let your penis — or your lover's penis — become a French fry: don't consume hydrogenated oils or fried foods. Trans fats are even worse for your arteries than saturated fats. Most baked products, despite their reassuring "No Trans Fats" labels, are laden with hidden trans fats produced when hydrogen is added to vegetable oil (changing it from a liquid to a solid). A baked product can still carry a "No Trans Fats" label, according to U.S. Food and Drug Administration regulations, if the amount of trans fats is below a certain arbitrary threshold that has no relationship to your health. With this piece of information in place,

the absolute worst meal for your sex life becomes a bacon cheeseburger with fries and a milkshake, followed by a dessert of baked trans-fats cookies.

4. Soy products. Some studies have shown soy helps to reduce cholesterol, but the downside is that soy foods imitate the female sex hormone, estrogen. Consuming large quantities of soy can flood your body with estrogen, and this can have a health impact on both sexes. It can feminize men, resulting in a lower sex drive and impotence, and it can produce a range of health effects in women, from an elevated risk of some diseases to increased production of testosterone, which is the female body's response to the presence of too much estrogen.

EXERCISE:
DETOX YOUR BODY, ENERGIZE YOUR SEXUALITY

Everyone who stays at the Hippocrates Health Institute as a guest, whether they enter our one-week, two-week, or three-week program, has an opportunity to detox their body fat and organs of synthetic chemical toxins. This is a necessary step in unburdening their immune system so that healthy cells can be produced to help regenerate and heal their body.

Given the toxic onslaught that we all face during a normal life, seeking protection for our sexual health to ensure lifelong sexual vitality requires that we periodically detox ourselves. Our Hippocrates program uses a synergistic approach to detoxification. We combine exercise, far-infrared saunas, a plant-based diet, fasting, specific supplements, colon hydrotherapy, therapeutic massage, pure water, and wheatgrass juice.

Most people have neither the interest nor the time to regularly undertake this complete detox regimen, incorporating all elements of our program. There are ways, however, to combine these detox techniques to effectively keep your body protected from the toxins that can ravage your sex life.

You might, for instance, combine an exercise routine with a sauna afterward, and take one of our recommended supplements to achieve good results. Or you might learn how to practice colon cleansing on your own, along with using purified water and wheatgrass juicing.

Here is a brief description of each of the eight detox techniques and how they benefit you:

1. Exercise. When we engage in vigorous exercise at least five times a week, our lungs and skin excrete some of the chemicals stored in our body. Exercise also facilitates blood flow, helping to keep veins and arteries open for maximum sensitivity of the sex organs.

2. Far-infrared saunas. These saunas produce high energy rather than just the high heat of conventional saunas, and their energy penetrates more deeply into body tissues to help release toxins. They are best used after vigorous exercise has opened your pores. If you don't have access to a far-infrared sauna at a gym or health spa, use a conventional sauna.

3. Fasting. We recommend one twenty-four-hour fast a week, drinking only pure water and green juices, including wheatgrass juice, to accelerate detoxification. Fasting helps to leach chemicals out of body fat. But do not fast if you have a blood sugar disorder or if you are experiencing a physical impairment that leaves you gaunt or weak.

4. Supplements. Our recommended supplement for detox is chlorella, a green algae that helps the body to rid itself of heavy metals and radiation effects. Other important detox supplements include cayenne pepper, capsicum, garlic, and edible green clay.

5. Colon hydrotherapy. Periodically cleansing the large intestine of

compacted waste also contributes to cleaning the body of toxins. Colon irrigation, whether done by a professionally trained colon hydrotherapist or performed on your own at home, can boost your energy level and with it your sexual vitality.

6. Therapeutic drainage massage. This detox massage of the lymph glands helps to reduce congestion in the body and strengthens the immune system. A certified massage therapist can perform this technique for you.

7. Pure water. Because our bodies are so dependent on water to flush out toxins, it is imperative that the water we use is pure so we don't further contribute to our toxicity. Don't drink tap water, which usually contains chlorine and fluoride, and can also be contaminated with numerous synthetic chemicals that water treatment plants cannot remove. Beware of most bottled water brands, especially Aquafina and Dasani, which are just recycled tap water. Purchase your own water purification system that uses advanced technology, and use it to filter the water you drink.

8. Wheatgrass and green drink juice. Almost pure chlorophyll, wheatgrass juice is effective in cleaning out the arteries, flushing out toxins, and assisting bone marrow to generate new cells. Sprouted wheatgrass is rich in phytochemicals, which help to protect us against physical degeneration and diseases.

Nourish Your Sexuality

*I think people should be free to engage
in any sexual practices they choose;
they should draw the line at goats though.*

— Singer Elton John

Infertility Sometimes Can Be Conquered

When a Stanford University oncologist informed thirty-two-year-old Andrea that the experimental cancer drug combination she was taking "will probably make you sterile," Andrea's lifelong dream of being a mother seemed to vanish in the face of her struggle against stage 4 Hodgkin's disease.

Since the age of sixteen, growing up on a dairy farm in Wisconsin, Andrea had experienced a recurring vivid dream in which she walked hand in hand with a little blond-haired boy who she sensed was her own future son. Now that cancer of the lymphatic system had infiltrated both lungs, her doctors wanted her to undergo chemotherapy, followed by a bone marrow transplant and radiation, in addition to a cocktail of seven experimental drugs. There was no doubt in anyone's mind that sterility would result from this treatment regimen.

"I knew that I had to put away my dreams of giving birth," Andrea told us during a visit to the Hippocrates Health Institute. "It was a huge feeling of loss. I'm the youngest of ten children, and I had always wanted a big family of my own. But my first concern had to be my own survival."

A friend gave Andrea a health book that mentioned our institute and our work with cancer patients. "I did the chemotherapy and the combination of seven experimental drugs. But the bone marrow transplant and radiation just didn't feel right for me. It was a strong intuitive feeling. So I decided to attend the three-week Hippocrates program. When I told my doctors, they tried to discourage me, saying the program was voodoo and pseudoscience."

With financial assistance from her future husband, Andrea entered Hippocrates and began eating right, meditating, exercising, and detoxing her body, filling it with raw living foods and juices. "By the second week, I could feel changes in my body, and I had so much energy that I felt like I was sixteen years old again. By the third week, I noticed the nagging pain in my vertebrae had disappeared. The tumor was no longer pressing against my spine."

When Andrea returned to Stanford for x-rays and an examination, her physicians were baffled by what they found. Not only had Andrea's tumor not grown and spread, as they had predicted, but it had diminished in size. "I don't know what to make of this," the chief oncologist confessed to Andrea. "You've given me reason to pause."

Six months passed, and the unexpected happened again: Andrea got pregnant, despite her doctor's prediction that she would be sterile from the drugs. Andrea's eyes tear up when she recalls how her hopes were realized. She gave birth to a blond-haired boy who resembled the one in her recurring dream, a birth she credits to the pure-foods diet that she integrated into her life.

Above the buffet counter at Hippocrates hangs a collection of eighteen baby photos showing some of the many children who have been born to women previously diagnosed as infertile, yet who gave birth after adopting the Hippocrates program. Some of these women had tried to conceive for decades.

Why are infertility statistics so high today? Surveys indicate that anywhere from 12 percent up to 33 percent of all couples are unable to conceive a child through natural means. Falling sperm counts are part of the problem. In the past half century, average sperm counts have fallen 40 percent, a substantial decline. Widespread exposure to synthetic chemicals that mimic estrogen, found in pesticides, foods, and personal care products, have feminized the reproductive capacity of many men.

Another factor in male infertility may be drugs intended to prolong sexual enjoyment. A 2007 study in the journal *Fertility and Sterility* studied human sperm in vitro and found that sildenafil, the chemical name for Viagra, causes sperm to prematurely release enzymes that facilitate penetration of the egg. As a result, many sperm that reach a woman's egg are unable to fertilize it if the man has taken Viagra in the preceding twenty-four hours.[1]

Another factor affecting male fertility is the expanding use of antidepressants. Two Cornell University Medical Center scientists reported in *New Scientist* magazine in September 2008 that in healthy men given paroxetine — sold as Paxil or Seroxat — an average of 30 percent of their sperm cells exhibited DNA fragmentation after just four weeks of antidepressant use, thus damaging the men's ability to father a child.[2]

The Overlooked Role of Nutrients in Fertility

Three decades ago, Dr. Henry G. Bieler's book *Dr. Bieler's Natural Way to Sexual Health* had this to say about the link between nutrition and sexual health: "Every area concerning human sexuality has been intensively investigated, except the role of nutrition and how it affects a person's sex life. I have proven in countless cases that improper diet causes damage to and malfunction of the sex organs, and that prescribing an individual proper diet leads to restoration of the male's virility and the return of feeling to the female's genital area."[3]

Dr. Stephen Holt, president of the Illinois College of Physicians and Surgeons, in his 1999 book *The Sexual Revolution*, also called nutrients a key to sexual vitality: "In my own clinical experience, I have seen individuals reverse sexual problems by balancing their diet and taking well selected dietary supplements. Certainly they may have changed their lifestyle in other ways to enhance sexual function, but good nutrition is the foundation for continuing good sex."[4]

Still another expert on nutrients and sexual health, Dr. Morton Walker, wrote in his 1994 book *Sexual Nutrition* about the effects on the male body of just one essential nutrient: zinc. He pointed out that the body of an average-weight twenty-year-old male normally contains 2.2 grams of zinc, most of it in the testes. If a young man has less than this amount of the mineral, it is unlikely that he would feel much of a sexual urge or be able to sustain an erection, much less produce enough semen to successfully impregnate a woman.[5]

Our Recommended Natural Alternatives to Fertility Drugs

- Cauliflower and other foods containing high levels of vitamin B
- Ginger in various forms as tea and spice for food
- Ginseng for male infertility
- Guava and other foods with high vitamin C for male infertility
- Spinach and other high-zinc-content foods for poor sperm quality
- Sunflower seeds and other foods containing the amino acid arginine
- Bottle gourd and other herbs containing choline
- Raspberry leaf tea
- Herbal formulas for female infertility (recipes with herb combinations)
- Herbal formulas for male infertility (Chinese herb recipes)

Did You Know?

Male Sexual Abstinence Undermines Fertility

If you are part of a couple trying to conceive a child, you should know that the longer the man goes without ejaculating, the less fertile his semen will become.

Evidence for this first began accumulating in the early 1990s, when studies done by medical teams in Norway and France uncovered the effects abstinence has on a range of semen health characteristics. After just ten days of abstinence, the motility of semen — their ability to swim upstream, so to speak, which is essential to egg fertilization — was found to be significantly reduced. "Lengthy sexual abstinence was found to affect all semen characteristics," reads a 1994 study in the *International Journal of Fertility & Menopausal Studies*, and semen "motility and normal morphology decreased significantly with duration of abstinence."[6]

A 2005 study in the journal *Fertility & Sterility* confirmed the earlier findings after testing 5,983 sperm samples. The study authors advise all couples seeking to conceive that men "not exceed 10 days of sexual abstinence" before engaging in procreative sexual activity.[7]

If you still aren't convinced by the evidence, another study, in 2009, should dispel any doubts. Australian researchers reported to a conference of the European Society for Human Reproduction and Embryology that eight of every ten men tested showed a 12 percent drop in sperm DNA damage after seven days if they had ejaculated every day.[8] This finding supports the idea that the longer sperm live in the testes, the more likely they are to develop DNA damage because of attacks by free radicals, those small reactive molecules that cause cell damage and death.

All of which is to say, having lots of sexual activity, preferably daily, around the time a woman is ovulating raises the chances of successful impregnation.

Diet Can Energize Your Sexual Health

A woman from New York who was a guest at Hippocrates came to us for counseling. She had been with her husband for twenty years and had three children with him, but the husband had lost interest in sexual intimacy about two years earlier. She immediately suspected this was a sign that he was being unfaithful.

Based on her descriptions of her husband, it became clear that there were other factors involved, not infidelity. His mother had died around the time he lost interest in sex. He had also lost his job, which meant he perceived that his manhood had been diminished. Then he suffered a heart attack, probably from the stress of everything that had happened.

Her perception had been that his change in sexual interest had little to do with her. While that was true, she hadn't factored in that he had lost desire as a result of the psychological blows. The more pressure she put on him sexually, the more she pushed him away. Once she got him on the Hippocrates diet and he began seeing a counselor to address his issues, everything changed, and they had more intimacy in their marriage than ever before.

Natural nutrients to energize sexuality can take some surprising forms beyond food itself. Consider these:

- There is a biological reason for the desire to engage in oral sex. It involves the antimicrobial actions of certain body fluids. The emotional underpinning, however, goes back to suckling at our mother's breast. But how many of us were breastfed? Some of us did not have this early urge fulfilled, and this lack might enhance the desire for oral sex.
- Even if a person is moderately sick, we would still encourage that person to attempt sexual intimacy because it helps to put them back into the psychological zone of vitality, which is important to recovery. If you don't use your sexuality, it becomes like a rusty wheel; you need to lubricate it with practice to get the sex hormones flowing again and to get the right combinations of muscle groups performing again. Never get off the sex bike as you mature. Keep riding.

Raw Foods Enhance Sexual Vitality

We conducted a survey of Hippocrates guests and employees — four couples and four singles — to gauge how a raw foods diet affects sexual vitality. Here are some of the responses we got in the interviews.

Jaime, fifty-five, and John, forty-two, had been married for fifteen years, and both commented they felt the diet enhanced their sexuality and overall health. "I've gone into menopause, but this diet has made it easier because I have more energy to work with," said Jaime, who described herself as eating a 70 percent raw food diet. "Sex was a release of tension for us in the beginning of our relationship," added John, "but now it's more healthy and nurturing. My body now craves wheatgrass juice, which gives me more desire." Jaime expanded on that theme: "Intensity increases because we feel everything. The energy we feel is amazing, and all of our senses are heightened on this diet."

Renee, fifty-three, and Stephan, thirty-eight, married in 1998 and consider themselves to be 90 percent raw. "My senses have been sharpened greatly by this diet, and I have a clarity of thought like I never had as a young person," commented Stephan, who lost sixty-five pounds after adopting raw foods. Though Renee didn't feel that the diet had changed her sexual desire or arousal levels in any obvious way, she did believe "the big change for me has been in the head. The diet allows me to remain healthy despite my hormones having taken a dive. I've also noticed that people on the Hippocrates diet are calmer, more understanding, and kind to one another, which may help to create more sexual intimacy."

Jimmy, fifty-six, and Frances, thirty-two, had been together just five months when they were interviewed, so the passion that flows from a new relationship must be factored into their perceptions. Both noticed a big difference in their sensations of desire, arousal, intensity of orgasm, and sexual stamina and performance after dropping meat and dairy products from their diets. Jimmy lost thirty pounds and hadn't been sick in the past seven years, while Frances reported that she no longer needed an inhaler for the asthma that had previously hospitalized her when she ate a conventional diet. "The raw food lifestyle has made a tremendous difference in my sexual energy and desire and arousal," said Jimmy. "We're both always horny now." Frances believed the biggest difference the diet made for her was that "I have the happiness that helps my sexuality to be expressed in a healthy way."

Kenneth, forty-four, and Pamela, forty-three, had married several years earlier, after meeting at Hippocrates. Kenneth had been a chef and owner of his own restaurant in Baltimore. He became a vegan at age forty, then went 90 percent raw, which "produced an immediate increase in my energy level. While eating this way and being married to Pamela, the length of time I can perform sexually has gone way up and my overall sexual satisfaction level is much higher." Pamela related how "I feel more vital on this diet and have more freedom to feel and express myself sexually. My senses are heightened in this committed and loving relationship."

Forty-nine-year-old Sherry is a divorced Long Island native who suffered multiple hormonal deficiencies and excruciating menstrual cycles during the years she ate meat and dairy products. She would experience fatigue and had no sexual desire at all for two weeks out of every month. She began to change her diet to become a vegetarian, then a vegan, and finally adopted an 80 percent raw diet. "During this process, the awful effects of my menstrual cycle got much better, but each time I went back to dairy products there was an instantaneous negative impact on my menstruation and desire levels," she told us. "Once I became raw, my energy level made a turnaround. I'm more sexually aware now, with more intense orgasms and a healthier libido. I've even had multiple orgasms for the first time in my life."

Eunice came to work at Hippocrates in 2001, shortly after being diagnosed with type 2 diabetes and high blood pressure. This sixty-four-year-old native of Jamaica adopted a mostly raw foods diet and experienced a remarkable improvement in her health. "I started feeling younger, stronger, and more vibrant. My insulin levels and blood pressure became normal again, and I discarded all of my medications. On the diet I became more sexually responsive, and my husband was very appreciative.

I started thinking about sex again, whereas before I had been pushing it away. I can testify that this diet will improve your sex life and improve the quality of your relationships."

A forty-nine-year-old physician from New York who makes frequent visits to Hippocrates, Dr. Sampson, had taken on a 100 percent raw diet that made him feel "more desirable and more confident, and that rolls over into my sexual vitality. I'm more sluggish and less sexually voracious on cooked foods. I broke down and had a hamburger with my children not long ago. I had sex that evening, after eating the hamburger, and I could clearly tell that I wasn't up to my usual standards of arousal and stamina and performance. I choose the foods I ingest much more consciously than ever before in my life because I know they will have an effect on my energy levels and libido."

Fifty-four-year-old Robyn grew up in New York feeling that having sex with multiple partners was a way of being loved and desired. Later in life, she began to shed the unhealthy relationships that were based on nothing but great sex, though her libido continued to burn brightly right through the age when most women experience menopause. "When you go raw, an incredible amount of honesty comes with that," she explained to us. "I still enjoy masturbating and sometimes please myself twice a day. It builds my immune system. I have more intense and even multiple orgasms since going raw. Being passionate in life and about life is just as important as being passionate in bed with another person."

Nutrients Essential to Sexual Health

B-Complex Vitamins

Action: These relax all systems in the body and are important to the production of hormones in both men and women. They are also builders of the T-cell and the B-cell in the immune system, both of which direct white blood cells in their jobs, including sex hormone creation.

Food sources: Sprouted grains of all types, uncooked whole-grain breads.

Beta-Carotene (Vitamin A)

Action: This one is best known for the positive effect it has on eye and skin health. It also plays a vital role in the production of sex hormones. It strengthens the mucus membranes, prevents atrophy of the genitals, and increases sperm count. The strength and numbers of white blood cells intensify with the absorption of this vitamin, and white blood cells are essential to the production of sex hormones.

Food sources: Leafy green sprouts (all varieties), collard greens, beet greens, kale, spinach, broccoli, cabbage, watermelon, cantaloupe, edible weeds such as dandelion, citrus fruits, mangos, papayas, persimmons, red and other colorful peppers, all squash, lettuce; root vegetables such as sweet potato, yams, carrots, jicama.

Calcium

Action: This is central to the development of bones and teeth, but it has also been linked to cellular health. When cells are healthy, they heighten sensitivity, a necessary ingredient for sexual pleasure. Calcium is also important to circulation to the genitalia.

Food sources: All leafy green vegetables, sprouts, every form of sprouted bean (excluding soy and black beans), the entire cabbage family, broccoli, kale, lentils, sea vegetables, wheatgrass juice, turnip greens, Swiss chard.

Choline

Action: Part of the B vitamin complex, it is essential to circulatory activity, blood cell development, and neurological function. It's important to have adequate amounts to regulate brain cell activity to balance mood, heighten happiness, and increase the potential for imagination.

Food sources: Avocados; sprouted beans (excluding soy and black beans), with an emphasis on sprouted garbanzo beans; lentils; peas and green-pea sprouts; the cabbage family, including Brussels sprouts, cauliflower, kale, broccoli, cabbage.

Essential Fatty Acids

Action: These are directly linked to every cell in the human body. They're the primary fuel for all cells. They are essential for sexual desire, sensitivity, and pleasure. The average person's diet includes less than 20 percent of the necessary essential fatty acids.

Food sources: Germinated nuts, seeds, grains, and beans. They should always be taken from a vegetarian/vegan source (fish oil becomes rancid within twenty-four hours and acts as a carcinogen). The best supplemental sources are walnuts and their oil, hemp and its oil, and flax and its oil. Preferable, too, are sprouted seeds, such as chia sprouts, which have oils that are more accessible to body cells.

Iron

Action: This red blood cell nutrient allows the absorption and transportation of oxygen to occur at the intercellular level throughout the systems of the body. Consistent usable iron is important to the skeletal structure and organs. As people age in an unhealthy way, lack of iron contributes to sexual dysfunction.

Food sources: Fruits such as peaches, apricots, and plums; beans such as lima, fava, white, navy, and pinto; sprouts such as pea greens, sunflower greens, and flaxseed; edible weeds such as lambsquarter and dandelion; pumpkin seeds; wheatgrass juice; sea vegetables; watercress; parsley.

Magnesium

Action: It's the muscle relaxant mineral, and every organ depends upon it for function. It also helps to maintain optimal prostate function and to prevent vaginal dryness due to hormonal weakness.

Food sources: Raw almonds, filberts, macadamia nuts; fruits such as peaches, bananas, persimmons; beans such as kidney, lentil, fava; buckwheat sprouts; sesame seeds; all forms of winter and summer squash; wheatgrass juice; spelt juice.

Niacin (Vitamin B3)

Action: This vitamin is important to the circulation of human blood. It allows blood flow to all organ and glandular systems and increases cellular activity, heightening sensitivity during the sexual experience. There are cases in which erectile dysfunction has been remedied in the short term by whole-food niacin supplementation.

Food sources: Avocados, green-pea sprouts, buckwheat sprouts, artichoke, kale, spinach; fruits such as watermelon, cantaloupe, and casaba melon. (Eating sprouted seeds intensifies the amount of niacin present.)

Pantothenic Acid (Vitamin B5)

Action: Necessary for hormone creation in both sexes.

Food sources: Asparagus, avocados, lentils, sprouted peas, sprouted quinoa, sprouted amaranth, cabbage, broccoli, broccoli sprouts, cauliflower, and fruits such as mangos, papayas, kiwis, guavas.

Pyridoxine (Vitamin B6)

Action: Another important activator of hormonal development. Both male and female testosterone levels depend upon this vitamin.

Food sources: Apples, pears, sprouted barley, sprouted spelt, sprouted wheat, weeds such as persling, aloe vera, all forms of lettuce, sesame and sunflower seeds and their sprouts, sweet potatoes.

Selenium

Action: This antioxidant is the most powerful immune system–boosting nutrient known today. White blood cells, the most prolific part of the immune system, are benefited by consistent amounts of selenium. Deficiencies today are most often caused by its absence in nonorganic farming soil. Selenium supplements may be necessary to ensure adequate amounts.

Food sources: Barley grass, kamut grass, pea greens, fenugreek sprouts, Brazil nuts, cabbage, Brussels sprouts, maitake and shiitake mushrooms, all seaweeds, spinach, ripe organic tomatoes, yellow and orange winter squash.

Vitamin B12

Action: A nutrient most lacking in modern diets, it is central to brain neuron health and nervous system strength. Its deficiency results in grave reduction of bodily functions, including those of the genitalia. Imagination and sexual desire both depend on this nutrient.

Food sources: Supplements with bacterial forms of B_{12}.

Vitamin D

Action: Deficiency is widespread in the population. This essential nutrient regulates moods and the protection of cells against mutagenic factors. It's also important for the development of all cells, including white blood cells, and must be part of every sexually healthy person's diet. Sun exposure for thirty minutes in both the early and late day is crucial several times weekly.

Food sources: Shiitake mushrooms (dry), chicory weed.

Vitamin E

Action: It is best known in the world of nutrients as a sex vitamin. Research has shown that it increases libido for both sexes and heightens desire, sensitivity, and longevity. It addresses symptoms of hormonal deficiencies due to the aging process and enhances sexual functions. It's best if vitamin E–rich foods are consumed two to three hours before sexual activity.

Food sources: Leafy green vegetables, avocados, blackberries, raspberries, gooseberries, huckleberries, most nuts excluding cashews and peanuts, sunflower green sprouts, fenugreek sprouts, alfalfa sprouts, chia sprouts, sweet potatoes, yams, carrots.

Did You Know?

Light Therapy May Improve Your Sexual Functioning

We all have heard that vitamin D absorbed through our skin from sunlight is important to overall health, but did you know that light interacts with the pineal gland in our heads to affect our sex drive?

A team of Italian researchers writing in a 2009 issue of *Psychotherapy and Psychosomatics* reported the results of a study involving a group of volunteers ages thirty-nine to sixty who had a diagnosis of low sex drive, sexual arousal disorder, or orgasmic disorder. These test subjects were randomly assigned to either a light treatment group or a placebo group. The bright light group had daily exposure to a white fluorescent lightbox fitted with an ultraviolet filter, whereas the placebo group had reduced light exposure.

After two weeks, the volunteers rated their sexual satisfaction levels on a scale of 1 to 10. In the researchers' words, "a significant improvement" in sexual satisfaction was observed in the light therapy group versus no improvement in the placebo group. The reason for this improvement seems to be the interaction between the pineal gland and intense light, which might suggest we need proper exposure to natural sunlight to enhance our sexual functioning.[9]

Zinc

Action: Zinc is another essential nutrient for immune system function and is best known for prostate health and clitoris sensitivity. Zinc deficiencies are widespread today due to stress levels. It is the only nutrient clinically proven to lessen the symptoms of cold and flu. It also plays a central role in the creation of hormones.

Food sources: Mung bean sprouts, pumpkin seed sprouts, leafy green vegetables, bee pollen, flower pollen, wheatgrass, spelt grass.

Did You Know?

There Are Clear Links among Diet, Coronary Disease, and Frigidity

Sexual frigidity in women, defined as partial or complete inability to be aroused sexually or to achieve orgasm, is higher in those with coronary artery disease than in those of any other health category.

The first major medical study showing this link came in 1976, in *Psychosomatic Medicine*, which made note of estimates that "the percentage of women who never or rarely have orgasm lies between 25% and 40%." Some of that percentage can be attributed to factors other than coronary artery disease, but many of the coronary artery cases are linked to orgasm problems.[10]

Numerous studies have subsequently shown that just as a high-fat, toxic diet plays havoc with male sexual function by narrowing the genital arteries, so, too, does this sort of diet narrow the genital arteries of women, directly contributing to arousal and orgasm problems.

The Problem with Oysters and Chocolate

Although oysters are well known as a source of zinc, they are better known as a toxic food. Even in the Bible, people are warned not to eat shellfish. They are the scavengers of the ocean and absorb all its poisons. There is more toxic pollution in the oceans than ever before in human history, including carcinogens that run off from the industrial and pharmaceutical industries. Any zinc benefit that would be gained from eating oysters would be far outweighed by the toxic effects of the synthetic chemicals and parasites found in oysters. (You may also want to refer to our upcoming book *Killer Fish* for more details on the health problems associated with an aquatic-based nonplant diet.)

Chocolate has received a lot of propaganda mileage for its phytochemical benefits, but it has a very high fat content, and most chocolate on the market is permitted by law to contain rat droppings of up to 10 percent of volume. Rats are attracted to the cocoa beans as they are transported via freighters. Chocolate has negative effects on the liver and gallbladder, and for the little phytochemical benefit you gain, it causes far more problems that weaken the immune system.

Did You Know?

Sexual Fluids Taste Like What You Eat

If you're a woman (or man) and liberated in matters of body fluids, you've probably had the experience of finding the taste of some semen to be acidic, bitter, or overly salty. The reason is probably related to an unhealthy diet.

The same holds true for the taste and smell of a woman's vaginal fluids. If she eats a lot of meat daily, it's going to alter her natural taste in a way that doesn't always inspire ravenous behavior in a sexual partner.

Cleaner living makes for a cleaner sexual dining experience. For tastier vaginal and prostate secretions, try consuming any food that's naturally high in chlorophyll. These include parsley, wheatgrass, and watercress.

Natural sugars from the body can be excreted in high levels into semen and vaginal juices if you eat pineapple or drink pineapple juice. Cranberry juice is also recommended.

By all anecdotal accounts, both male and female vegetarians taste better than meat eaters. So avoid junk food, processed foods, meat, and dairy if you want to be a taste treat.

EXERCISE: KEGEL YOUR WAY TO SEXUAL VITALITY

The effects of sexually nourishing foods and nutrients can be further enhanced and a synergy created if your exercise program includes a simple technique called the Kegel.

Pronounced "KAY-gul" and named after the doctor who developed it, Arnold Kegel, this exercise was originally introduced in 1948 as a way to control incontinence in women after childbirth. Its medical use was later expanded to include men who experienced urinary incontinence after prostate surgery.

An unexpected benefit of Kegel exercises proved to be an improvement in sexual functioning in both men and women. Women with persistent problems reaching orgasm and men with erection-firmness difficulties generally report improvement after a month of practicing Kegels, which basically involves repeatedly flexing the pelvic floor muscles. But anyone can benefit from the technique in ways that intensify sexual pleasure. It's especially helpful to people in their fifties and beyond who want to maintain youthful sexual vigor.

Find the Pelvic Muscles

According to the Mayo Clinic (MayoClinic.com), the best way to find these muscles is to practice stopping the flow of urine while urinating. Another technique is to insert a finger into the vagina or the anus and practice tightening around the finger. You'll feel the pelvic muscles rise as you tighten them, then fall again as you relax.

Practice the Exercise

Several times a day, contract your pelvic muscles and hold the contraction for three seconds, then relax for three seconds. Repeat this process ten times. It's a versatile exercise that you can do most anywhere. You can do it while you're driving, sitting at a desk or computer, sitting in a chair reading, or lying down.

Keep increasing the time you contract and hold the muscles. But do this with an empty bladder. Work your way up to ten seconds for each contraction and hold. As you contract and hold, don't hold your breath. Continue breathing freely and normally. And make certain that the only muscles you're contracting are in the pelvic area.

Women can also practice the exercise by inserting a vaginal cone or rubber dildo into their vagina or anus and contracting the muscles around it. This practice has the added benefits of tightening the vagina in women who have given birth, and giving women more sphincter muscle control to use in gripping and pleasuring the penis during anal intercourse.

For men, contracting the anal sphincter muscle with regularity may also bestow the benefit of experiencing orgasms without ejaculation, which is a goal of tantric practices.

You will probably need to make Kegel exercises a lifelong practice to receive long-term rewards.

Did You Know?

Semen Absorption Is Good for Mental Health

If you've overcome your resistance to contact with another person's sexual fluids, you might be heartened to know that absorbing semen is good for your mood.

Semen acts as an antidepressant if absorbed vaginally or anally, according to a 2002 study in the journal *Archives of Sexual Behavior*, which tracked the moods of 293 women. Those who used condoms during intercourse were much more likely to suffer from depression or suicidal impulses than women who absorbed their partners' semen.[11]

These results were confirmed in a similar but larger study that examined mood-altering hormones in semen, including testosterone, estrogen, follicle-stimulating hormone, luteinizing hormone, prolactin, and several prostaglandins. Many of these have been measured at higher levels in women's blood within hours of absorbing semen.[12]

Evolutionary biologists speculate that men whose semen better enhanced a sex partner's long-term mood may have had an evolutionary advantage over other men in attracting sexual mates, which might explain why the mood-altering ability of semen persists until this day.

Still another unheralded benefit of absorbing semen through oral-genital contact is the retarding of tooth decay. That's right! Semen contains zinc, calcium, and other minerals that have demonstrated abilities to fight tooth degeneration.

Twelve Sexually Stimulating Recipes

The next time you anticipate or plan an intimate encounter, try preparing one of these meals and see if you can tell a difference in your and your partner's sexual desire and performance. (Our thanks to the Hippocrates Health Institute kitchen staff, especially chef Ken Blue and his wife, Pam, for preparing these recipes.)

We have taken the ten nutrients that most powerfully enhance libido and desire and combined them in the following recipes, which are designed to heighten the production of sex hormones via their synergistic interactions.

These nutrients are found in sexual vitality superfoods, including açaí fruit, avocados, Brazil nuts, broccoli, collard greens, figs, goji berries, green coconuts, kale, mustard greens, noni fruit, plums, spinach, colorful vegetables, sprouts, Swiss chard, walnuts, herbs, and medicinal mushrooms.

Broccoli Shiitake Arame with Sesame Ginger Dressing

Yield: 4–6 servings

Dressing

    ¼ cup fresh lemon juice

    1½-inch piece fresh ginger root, roughly chopped

    ¼ cup raw sesame oil

    1 large clove garlic

    1 tablespoon kelp powder

    Pinch of cayenne pepper

    Bragg Liquid Aminos

    1 large bunch or 2 small bunches broccoli, chopped into ½-inch florets

    2 Japanese shiitake mushrooms

    ¼ cup shredded daikon

    ¼ cup shredded carrot

    1 cup arame (see note below), soaked until soft (about 45 minutes) and drained

To make the dressing, in a blender, combine the lemon juice, ginger, sesame oil, garlic, kelp powder, and cayenne. Blend on high until smooth. Season to taste with Bragg Liquid Aminos.

In a medium bowl, combine the broccoli, shiitake, daikon, carrot, and arame. Add about ½ cup of the dressing. Toss to mix thoroughly. Add the remaining dressing, if you like, and serve. Store any unused dressing in an airtight container in the refrigerator for up to a week.

Note: Arame is a shredded, dried sea vegetable that is typically available at natural food stores or Asian markets.

Creamed Spinach

Yield: 4–6 servings

Sauce

> 3 tablespoons lemon juice
> 1½ cups pine nuts, soaked overnight at room temperature, drained, and rinsed
> 1½ teaspoons kelp powder
> 1 teaspoon oregano
> 5 ounces water
> 1½ cloves garlic
> Pinch of cayenne pepper
>
> 1 pound spinach, chopped in food processor with S blade
> 1 cup shredded yellow squash

In a blender, combine the sauce ingredients. Blend until creamy.

In a large bowl, pour the sauce over the spinach and toss to mix thoroughly. Top with the squash, and serve.

Sproutaghetti

Yield: 4–6 servings

> 4 red bell peppers, seeded and roughly chopped
> ½ red onion, roughly chopped
> 1 bunch fresh basil
> 2 cloves garlic, put through a garlic press
> 1 tablespoon Frontier Pizza Seasoning (see note below)
> ¼ cup extra virgin olive oil
> 1 teaspoon fresh lemon juice
> 1½ teaspoons kelp powder
> 1 tablespoon dried basil
> 1½ teaspoons dried oregano
> 1 teaspoon psyllium husk powder (optional; see note below)
> 8 cups bean sprouts
> Pitted sun-dried Greek black olives (optional)

In a food processor, combine the pepper, onion, fresh basil, garlic, pizza seasoning, olive oil, lemon juice, kelp powder, dried basil, and oregano, and process until smooth. If you prefer a thicker sauce, add the psyllium husk powder.

In a large bowl, pour the sauce over the bean sprouts and olives (if using), toss to mix thoroughly, and serve.

Note: Frontier Pizza Seasoning is our favorite brand of pizza seasoning, and it's available at many natural food stores. If you can't find it, substitute another brand of pizza seasoning. Psyllium husk powder is often available in bulk at natural food stores.

"Meaty" Cabbage

Yield: 2–4 servings

Dressing

> 3 tablespoons fresh lemon juice
> 1 small clove garlic
> 1 teaspoon kelp powder
> Pinch of cayenne pepper
> 6 tablespoons extra virgin olive oil
>
> 1 large head green cabbage, thinly sliced
> ¼ red onion, cut in short, thin slices

"Meaty" Mix

> 1½ cups walnut halves or pieces, soaked 8 to 10 hours at room
>   temperature and dehydrated
> ¼ teaspoon garlic powder
> 1 tablespoon Frontier Pizza Seasoning (see note page 118)
> 1 teaspoon Bragg Liquid Aminos

In a blender, combine the dressing ingredients and blend on high until smooth.

In a large bowl, combine the cabbage and onion. Pour the sauce on top and toss lightly. Let the mixture marinate for at least 1 hour.

In a food processor or blender, combine the "meaty" mix ingredients. Pulse until the mixture has the texture of cooked ground beef.

Add the "meaty" mix to the cabbage mixture, toss well, and serve.

Szechuan Mustard Greens

Yield: 2–4 servings

Dressing

    2 cups chopped seeded red bell pepper
    1 cup raw almond butter
    ½ cup chopped scallions
    ¼ cup chopped red beet
    1 tablespoon fresh lemon juice
    1 clove garlic
    1½ tablespoons kelp powder
    1 cup water
    1 tablespoon Bragg Liquid Aminos or nama shoyu (raw soy sauce)
    1½ teaspoons chopped fresh ginger root
    Cayenne pepper

    1 large or 2 small bunches mustard greens (or baby mustard greens, if available), chopped into bite-size pieces

To make the dressing, in a blender, combine the bell pepper, almond butter, scallion, beet, lemon juice, garlic, kelp powder, water, Bragg Liquid Aminos, and ginger. Blend until smooth, and season to taste with cayenne pepper (see note below).

In a large bowl, pour about half of the dressing over the mustard greens and toss to mix thoroughly. Add more dressing if you like, and serve. Store any unused dressing in an airtight container in the refrigerator for up to 5 days.

Note: Mustard greens vary greatly in their spiciness depending on freshness and variety. Taste the greens before adding the dressing. You may wish to use more or less cayenne in the dressing depending on how spicy the greens are. Also, for added crunch and flavor, try adding chopped almonds, bean sprouts, shredded carrots, or daikon.

Basily Broccoli Fennel

Yield: 2–4 servings

Dressing

>4 tablespoons fresh lemon juice
>1½ teaspoons kelp powder
>1 clove garlic
>1½ teaspoons herbes de Provence
>½ pound fresh basil leaf
>Pinch of cayenne pepper
>½ cup extra virgin olive oil
>
>1 large bunch or 2 small bunches broccoli, cut into small florets
>1 bulb fennel, thinly sliced
>¼ red onion, julienned
>½ red bell pepper, seeded and julienned
>½ cup chopped dehydrated Brazil nuts

In a blender, combine the dressing ingredients and blend until smooth. This will be a thick dressing with a good, strong basil flavor.

In a large bowl, combine the broccoli, fennel, onion, bell pepper, and Brazil nuts. Pour the dressing on top, toss thoroughly, and serve.

Lovin' Kale Beet Salad

Yield: 2–4 servings

Dressing

    ½ cup fresh lemon juice
    ½-inch piece fresh ginger root
    ½ cup sesame oil
    Pinch of cayenne pepper
    1 small clove garlic
    1 ½ teaspoons kelp powder
    ½ cup sauerkraut
    ¼ bunch dill

    2 bunches lacinato kale, stemmed and thinly sliced
    3 large beets, shredded

In a blender, combine the dressing ingredients and blend until smooth.

In a large bowl, massage the dressing into the kale until the kale is soft. Add the beets and toss thoroughly. Let marinate for at least 1 hour, and serve.

Cajun Collards with Pecans

Yield: 2–4 servings

Dressing

 2 red bell peppers, seeded and roughly chopped
 1 cup water
 1 large clove garlic
 1 tablespoon Frontier Pizza Seasoning (see note page 118)
 1 tablespoon fresh lemon juice
 2 drops liquid stevia extract, plus 1 more drop if needed
 1 teaspoon kelp powder
 1 cup raw sesame tahini

 2 bunches collard greens, stemmed and thinly sliced
 ¼ red onion, thinly sliced
 ½ cup dehydrated pecans, plus up to ½ cup more if needed

To make the dressing, in a blender, combine the bell pepper, water, garlic, pizza seasoning, lemon juice, stevia extract, and kelp powder. Blend until liquefied. Add the tahini and blend until creamy.

In a large bowl, massage about half of the dressing into the collards. Add more dressing if necessary to coat the greens and achieve the flavor you desire. Crumble the pecans on top of the greens. Add the onion, and stir to combine. Crumble more pecans on top if you like, and serve. Store any unused dressing in an airtight container in the refrigerator for up to 5 days.

Nikolai's Soup

Yield: 2–4 servings

¼ cup lemon juice

1-inch piece fresh ginger root, sliced

1 tablespoon Bragg Liquid Aminos, plus more as needed

2 cloves garlic

¼ teaspoon stevia powder or liquid

5 cups water

¼ cup sesame oil

½ bunch parsley

4 stalks celery

Pinch of cayenne pepper

1 cup shredded carrots

1 cup shredded parsnips

½ cup chopped dill

½ cup chopped scallions

2 avocados, pitted and diced

In a blender, combine the lemon juice, ginger, 1 tablespoon Bragg Liquid Aminos, garlic, stevia, water, sesame oil, parsley, celery, and cayenne. Blend until smooth. Season to taste with additional Bragg Liquid Aminos, if desired.

In a large bowl, combine the carrot, parsnip, dill, scallion, and avocado. Pour in the liquid from the blender, stir thoroughly, and serve.

Thai Coconut Curry Soup

Yield: 4–6 servings

2 cups shiitake mushrooms, sliced
2 tablespoons fresh lime or lemon juice, plus extra for shiitake
    mushrooms
2 cloves garlic
2-inch piece fresh ginger root, roughly chopped
1 teaspoon curry powder
1 cup fresh coconut meat
2 cups coconut water
2 cups water
2 scallions
1 avocado, halved and pitted
Pinch of cayenne pepper

Sprinkle shiitake mushrooms with lime or lemon juice and set aside.

In a blender, combine the 2 tablespoons lime or lemon juice, garlic, ginger, curry powder, coconut meat, coconut water, water, scallion, avocado, and cayenne. Blend until smooth. Add the shiitake, and serve.

Brazil Nut Milk

Yield: 4–6 servings

  2 cups Brazil nuts, soaked for 8 to 10 hours, drained, and rinsed
  5 cups water

In a blender, combine the Brazil nuts and water. Blend on high for 15 to 20 seconds. Strain through a nut/sprout bag or cheesecloth, and serve.

Note: This is great plain, or you can add goji berries, frozen bananas, cinnamon, or vanilla.

Hot Blend

Yield: approximately 1 cup

  ½ cup açaí berries
  ¼ cup goji berries
  ¼ cup blueberries

In a blender, combine açaí berries, goji berries, and blueberries. Blend on high for 30 seconds, and serve.

Enhance Your Sexuality

Sex is one of the nine reasons for reincarnation.
The other eight are unimportant.

— Comedian George Burns (1896–1996)

Channel Sexual Energy with Your Mind

Some things are better than sex, and some are worse,
but there's nothing exactly like it.

— Actor W. C. Fields (1880–1946)

Human sexuality is ordinarily channeled and released as a procreative act, to tranquilize yourself, or as a form of recreation. Sometimes it's a combination of these things. You might decide to tranquilize yourself to relieve stress, for instance, by having a bout of mindless recreational sex.

But what if we told you there was a fourth category of sexual expression and release, a mindful practice that few in the West have tried, an ancient technique so powerful that both men and women are said to experience multiple orgasms while engaged in it, enabling them to reach a transcendent state of spiritual bliss? This isn't just New Age mythmaking.

Sacred sexuality, better known as *tantra*, is how this sexual yoga practice has been introduced to westerners. The word *tantra* in Sanskrit, loosely translated, means "to weave." Its roots go back several thousand years to India's Hindu and Buddhist spiritual traditions, though it should be emphasized that tantra is not a religion in itself, and anyone from any religious background or belief system can find benefit from it.

As a practice, tantra has evolved into two "paths" — the "right-hand path," as it's called, refers to practitioners who use only yoga, meditation, mantra chanting, and related rituals to achieve a blissful, orgasmic state of consciousness, without sexual activity. The "left-hand path" of tantra actively uses sexuality as the vehicle for reaching spiritual states of consciousness by mindfully controlling orgasmic energy. To many western ears, talk about using sex with the intention of liberating spirit may sound scary and suspiciously like New Age jargon. But that may be because sexual tantric practices run so counter to repressive western attitudes about sex, and because western religious traditions have erected such stubborn boundaries between spirit and the pleasures of the flesh.

The website Tantra.com defines sacred sexuality as meditative and intimate lovemaking that can "prolong the act of making love and to channel, rather than dissipate, potent orgasmic energies moving through you, thereby raising the level of your consciousness."[1] When *tantrikas* (people who practice tantra) talk about bio-energy, they are referring to that electric current we feel coursing through our nervous system, which reaches its explosive peak during orgasm.

Tantra provides lessons in conscious intimacy to enable anyone to expand their potential for pleasure, though pleasure is not the ultimate goal of its practice. Tantric rituals between loving partners create a sort of container — an expanded comfort zone — that holds sexual energy just as a battery holds an electrical charge. These practices can bestow heightened control over sexual functioning for both men and women, and provide a way for couples to simultaneously overcome sexual dysfunctions — such as premature ejaculation in men and arousal problems in women — while elevating the sexual act to a new plane of spiritual experience. Tantra and the equally ancient Taoist sex instruction tradition from China are holistic strategies for using mindful sexuality as an approach to good health.

You can connect your heart and your partner's heart via the genitals through tantric exercises that intensify intimacy and passion. Here is one simple yet profound exercise you can try out the next time you are sexually intimate with someone you care about, either to establish a heart connection or to deepen one that already exists.

1. Sit facing each other, unclothed. Set a mood by turning off the lights or burning a few candles. If you play music, choose a slow and melodic instrumental, on low volume.
2. Place your left hand lightly over your partner's genitals, and have your partner do the same to you. Place your right hand lightly over your partner's heart, and have your partner do the same to you.
3. As you gaze into each other's eyes, take slow, deep breaths, and synchronize those breaths until you are both breathing in air and expelling it together.
4. Stay connected this way, keeping your mind as clear as possible of all thoughts, as you stay in the moment and absorb your partner's energy presence.
5. You can increase the hand pressure at the heart and genitals as a prelude to engaging in lovemaking. Or you can use this exercise as long-term foreplay for future intimacy in the hours or days ahead.

Conscious breathing is a tantric exercise that adds powerful energy to lovemaking, enabling you to maintain a high state of arousal. By practicing slow, rhythmic deep-belly breathing, punctuated by the release of sounds and movement, you harness sexual energy to make prolonged multiple orgasms and full-body orgasms possible.

One of our Hippocrates health-care employees, Theresa, a native of Pennsylvania, took a tantra weekend workshop in Florida at the age of twenty-seven that introduced her to the concept of sacred sexuality.

"Before the tantra workshop, I had to overcome my fear of exposing myself, not with nudity, but by revealing myself emotionally. I also had the fear of getting aroused in front of others. But I plunged ahead anyway because I understood that I'm a fearful person every day."

During the workshop, she learned breathwork and how to conduct energy movement within the body. Most important, she came to view tantra as one of the many doorways into sacred sexuality, a higher level of sexual expression that most cultures have forgotten. After the workshop, she had what she describes as a "sacred sexual breakthrough experience" while working with a shaman, an experience that made her even more conservative about whom she chooses to exchange sexual energy with. She took still another step in her personal evolution when she adopted a raw foods diet, which "became the foundation of allowing my mind to unlock and express the spiritual dimensions of sex."

Tantra can reignite a couple's sexual excitement, spirit of exploration, and creative intimacy. It can also provide, as it did with Theresa, an introduction to other forms of sacred sexuality. Life is (or should be) an adventure, and what better way to express it than by experiencing a sacred sexuality that brings intimacy and love right to the heart and center of a relationship? (Learn more about tantric sexual practices by consulting any of the books and websites that we have listed in the resources and bibliography.)

The Importance of Sex Rituals

Sacred sexuality takes multiple forms and embraces a range of religious and spiritual traditions that use ritual to channel sexual "energies," terminology that can refer to the life force and vitality as well as sexual desires and thoughts.

Within Orthodox Judaism, laws of family purity prescribe sexual rituals and behaviors based on whether they advance the purpose of holiness. One of our Hippocrates guests, Edith, the widow of a prominent Hasidic rabbi in New York, detailed for us how this works in practice.

Using the Torah as a guideline, Orthodox adherents maintain a separation of the sexes until marriage. Once married, a man doesn't touch a woman until she has completed her menstrual cycle each month. Sexual relations occur during two weeks of every month, with the two weeks of abstinence giving the couple time to intensify their desire for each other, which makes for a more potent and electric relationship when they are intimate, and also heightens the chances for successfully conceiving a child, if procreation is their goal.

When the Orthodox have sexual relations, Edith noted, "great significance is placed on a couple's thoughts. Only pure thoughts of love should be present, so that the divine presence of God joins them. If a man is thinking of a woman other than his wife when his seed enters his wife, or if he is thinking evil or impure thoughts, then the potential is there to affect the cellular level that will shape the child in a negative way."

Before going away on a business trip, an Orthodox man must unite with his wife if she isn't menstruating. "He is obligated to be intimate with his wife to make her feel secure and loved while he's gone. It's also good for the man so he doesn't spill his seed while away. These laws of family purity are all designed to keep marriages together and to keep love alive."

Edith pointed out that it's a myth that Orthodox couples are allowed to be intimate only through a hole cut in a sheet. "If a couple had relations while clothed, it would be considered more animalistic, so they are always unclothed. They should be in the dark and under the covers. It's all because of modesty and to elevate the act spiritually. Intimacy should always be a holy act. This joy is a gift from God. Holiness, purity, love, and respect are the bottom-line values for all of these Orthodox laws."

The fifty-year-old manager of the Hippocrates store, Christina grew up Irish Catholic in Washington, D.C., but later in life took another path toward sacred sexuality when she began practicing Buddhism. She had been quite inhibited as a teenager and young adult and never felt comfortable with her sexuality. "It was only my practice of Buddhism that loosened the inhibitions on my sexuality," she told us. "I had to work on my heart energy a lot and overcome the conditioning of my childhood. By opening my heart and having a determination to transform myself, I've created a sexual opening that is like a healing process."

Fifty-eight-year-old Gwen organized our first health educator program at Hippocrates decades ago, when the institute was still based in Boston. Since 1979, she has practiced Kundalini yoga, part of a spiritual path associated with the meditative tradition of tantra, in which sexuality is expressed through a meditative mind rather than just through physical release. This yogic practice is done by couples to align sexual energies with sacred experience.

She described for us what sacred sexuality means to her and her husband: "When you are in touch with the divine flow of energy and the intricate design of everything around us, and how it harmonizes and all comes together, you overflow with awe and gratitude. When you come into contact with someone who also knows that arena of energy, the union between male and female creates a new and more powerful level of intimacy. That experience of ecstasy is a precious gift to relationships. It unites us with the divine."

You can't have sexual intercourse that is spiritual or grounded in spirituality without it bringing some level of fulfillment and joy. We humans possess a biological drive to touch and have sexual relations, but most of us also want to express our spiritual nature through the sexual act.

It's a spiritual act, for example, when a child is conceived. That is God, the life force, and nature, however you perceive it, at work. The altered state that comes from the biochemical release and euphoria of orgasm has a spiritual overtone. It's like God's way of seducing us into perpetuating humanity.

We can even wonder and speculate about whether the personality and sex of a child are determined at conception based on the level of consciousness the couple shares at the moment of orgasm. We believe that sex is a gateway to godliness and spirituality, just as deep contemplation, meditation, and prayer are gateways into the realm of the divine.

Did You Know?

Orgasm Can Be Separated from Ejaculation

If you're like most people, you probably think that orgasm and ejaculation of semen are inseparable partners, like Siamese twins, in the male sexual experience. After all, how often do men have an orgasm that doesn't produce a seminal fluid eruption?

The answer might surprise you, especially if you've never experienced it or seen it happen. Not only can orgasm be separated from ejaculation in men, but men can have multiple orgasms just as some women do.

Ejaculation is a glandular reflex that occurs when a physiological threshold — the point of no return — is crossed and the prostate gland contracts to discharge seminal fluid.

Orgasm, on the other hand, is an emotional, energetic reflex that produces waves of physical sensation and involuntary muscular movements.

Taking control over your breath is the key to having an orgasm without triggering the reflex of ejaculation. The point of no return can be bypassed by substituting deep breathing exercises for the shallow chest breaths that usually accompany sexual activity. It takes practice, but any man can learn to do it. For women, there is an added benefit — their sex partners who master this practice can sustain intercourse for much longer periods of time.

To learn about how to use breathing to disengage ejaculation from orgasm, and how to experience multiple orgasms with this technique, consult the resources at the back of this book.

Natural Sex Boosters for Men and Women

Watermelon May Be the New Viagra

We've always known it to be a juicy fruit that's about 92 percent water, but until recently no one had any idea that the remaining 8 percent of content in watermelon is loaded with rich nutrients for sexual health.

Researchers at the Texas A&M Fruit and Vegetable Improvement Center reported findings in 2008 that watermelon has ingredients that deliver Viagra-like effects to the human body's blood vessels and could even help to increase libido.

Watermelon contains a phytonutrient — part of a family of naturally occurring compounds that trigger healthy reactions in the body. This phytonutrient is called citrulline, which the body converts to arginine, an amino acid that "works wonders on the heart and circulation system and maintains a good immune system," says Dr. Bhimu Patil, director of the Fruit and Vegetable Improvement Center.

Arginine boosts nitric oxide levels in the body, which relax blood vessels in the same way that Viagra does, so that erectile dysfunction can be treated and perhaps even prevented if enough watermelon is consumed. "Watermelon may not be as organ specific as Viagra," notes Patil, "but it's a great way to relax blood vessels without any drug side effects."

Citrulline is found in its highest concentrations in watermelon rinds, which, of course, few people eat. But scientists at Texas A&M are breeding new varieties of watermelon that will contain higher concentrations of citrulline in their watery flesh.

Another nutrient found at high levels in watermelon is lycopene, an antioxidant normally associated with tomatoes that helps to protect the human heart, prostate gland, and skin.[2]

Mother's Milk Is an Aphrodisiac

Throughout human history, virtually anything that grows, be it plant or animal, has been experimented with to determine whether it can make men and women sexually ravenous. One of the best aphrodisiacs, it turns out, may be in a place where no one thought to look.

A woman's breastmilk is not only a nutrient for babies; other women's exposure to it may enhance their own sex lives. Researchers at the University of Chicago ran an experiment in 2004 in which female volunteers smelled either pads worn by breastfeeding mothers or pads doused with a neutral solution. Women in relationships who absorbed the aroma of breastmilk experienced a 24 percent increase in sexual desire for their partners, while single women measured a 17 percent increase in desire. Women who sniffed the "neutral" pads reported no such enhancement of sexual desire.

The researchers speculated that breastmilk releases a sexual chemosignal that affects other women's moods when its scent is absorbed through the nose. This natural libido booster may be a byproduct of our evolutionary history. Chemosignals could have acted to stimulate sexual desire among groups of women to ensure the survival of population groups by raising birth rates.[3]

So if you want to naturally jump-start your libido, hang around lactating women for a while!

Nineteen Nourishing Aphrodisiac Foods

Many foods can nourish both your body and your sexuality. Mung bean sprouts, for example, which are known as Chinese bean sprouts, are the richest natural source of zinc, essential for testosterone building. Also nutrient rich are pumpkin seeds, preferably soaked and sprouted, which have the full spectrum of zinc that enhances dihydrotestosterone (DHT), which fosters testosterone development. Shiitake mushrooms, wheatgrass juice, and wheat sprouts are all helpful in the process of developing and maintaining testosterone.

Here are nineteen foods that can strengthen your libido:

Apricots and apricot pits: These contain abscisic acid (B17), which invigorates sexual hormones. For best results, consume up to fifteen apricot pits several hours before sexual intimacy. (Pits can be pulverized or powdered.)

Black raspberries (fruit and seeds): This phytochemical-rich food enhances both libido and sexual endurance. Consume ten black raspberries, or one tablespoon of their seeds, about two hours before being sexually intimate.

Dill: For women, this herb helps to increase egg production and the desire for intimacy.

Figs: Considered excellent stimulants of fertility, figs also enhance the secretion of pheromones. Eat up to five figs with your partner before intimacy.

Flower pollen: This is a white blood cell strengthener with aphrodisiac qualities. Take one tablespoon of it every morning for exceptional nutrition and increased libido.

Hibiscus: A gland stimulator; sip tea made from this flower before engaging in intimacy.

Jerusalem artichoke: An energy vegetable, but one without sugars. Take four ounces on the morning of any planned sexual intimacy.

Lentil sprouts: Minerals and vitamins in these sprouts help to stimulate hormones. Consume about three to five ounces an hour before intimate contact.

Lettuce: Iceberg lettuce contains an opiate that helps to activate sex hormones. Eat one bowl of organic iceberg lettuce three hours before intimacy.

Mulberries: Consume one or two handfuls of this phytonutrient-rich fruit, long valued as an aphrodisiac food, just before foreplay.

Nutmeg: Known for its effects on a woman's hormones; best if two to three tablespoons are consumed an hour before intimate contact.

Oat sprouts: The expression "sow your wild oats" comes from their reputation as an aphrodisiac that stimulates sexual vitality. Eat three to four ounces of uncooked oat sprouts about four hours before sexual relations.

Pea greens: Containing high levels of amino acids, these enhance red blood cell production and can sexually arouse males. Juice and drink two to four ounces an hour before intimacy. Eating pea greens in salad form may also provide sexual stimulation.

Infamous Sex Myth

Spanish Fly Makes You Horny

Maybe you're old enough to remember this urban folk legend.

A young man gives his virginal girlfriend a soda spiked with Spanish fly. He momentarily leaves her in his parked car. On his return, he finds her sexually aroused and frantically humping the car's gearshift, which she has impaled up her vagina.

For most females, this became a cautionary tale. For some boys, it was inspiration to rush out and find the nearest Spanish fly dealer.

As with many inflated legends, this one has a morsel of truth. Spanish fly does exist. It's a powder made from a species of Mediterranean beetle. When swallowed, it irritates the lining of the bladder and urethra, resulting in an inflamed clitoris in women. It can make those who consume it want to rub themselves, but only to relieve their discomfort.

Adverse reactions can go well beyond inflammation. Just a few milligrams of Spanish fly can permanently damage your kidneys. Heavier doses can result in coma or death.

Radicchio: Its mineral and trace mineral content helps to confer sexual endurance on both men and women. Eat two ounces about eight hours before sexual contact.

Spelt sprouts: These protein-rich grains contain high levels of vitamins and amino acids; try eating one cup two to four hours before intimacy to increase sexual endurance.

Tomato seeds: Sun-dried organic tomato seeds contain high levels of phytonutrients that invigorate the sex hormones. Consume two to three ounces about an hour before sex.

Watermelon-seed sprouts: White blood cell counts are increased by these complete proteins, which in turn enhance sexual vitality. Juice and drink six ounces before intimacy.

Yams: Both men and women experience elevated hormone levels after consuming raw yams, in either grated or sprouted form. Take three to six ounces about two hours before contact.

Zucchini: You can use it either juiced or raw, and these delightful summer squash enhance blood circulation and help both desire and performance. Eat about three ounces three hours before your anticipated sexual encounter.

Scientific Evidence for Natural Aphrodisiacs

Study 1: Nutmeg

Background: Many traditional cultures have used nutmeg to treat male sexual disorders for hundreds, if not thousands, of years. One study from India administered a 50 percent ethanolic extract of nutmeg to groups of male rats daily for seven days in the presence of female rats.

Findings: "The resultant significant and sustained increase in the sexual activity of normal male rats without any conspicuous adverse effects indicates that the 50% ethanolic extract of nutmeg possesses aphrodisiac activity, increasing both libido and potency."[4]

Study 2: Clove

Background: Since ancient times, the flower bud of *Syzygium aromaticum* (clove) has been used in India to treat male sexual disorders. In a research study, an extract of clove was given to male rats for seven days in the presence of female rats.

Findings: "The results indicated that the 50% ethanolic extract of clove produced a significant and sustained increase in the sexual activity of normal male rats, without any conspicuous gastric ulceration and adverse effects. Thus, the resultant aphrodisiac effectivity of the extract lends support to the claims for its traditional usage in sexual disorders."[5]

Study 3: Casimiroa Edulis Seed

Background: Thirty healthy male rats were fed either a *Casimiroa edulis* seed extract or sildenafil citrate, the active ingredient in Viagra, to compare the effectiveness of each.

Findings: Both groups of rats exhibited a heightened sexual activity, prompting the researchers to write, "Our work provides preliminary evidence that the seed extract possesses aphrodisiac activity and may be used as an alternative drug therapy to restore sexual functions."[6]

Study 4: Tribulus Terrestris

Background: Traditional Chinese and Indian systems of medicine have used this botanical to improve sexual functioning. In this study, both normal and castrated rats were administered the substance to test its aphrodisiac effects.

Findings: "These results were statistically significant. It is concluded that Tribulus Terrestris extract appears to possess aphrodisiac activity probably due to [the] androgen increasing property of TT."[7]

Study 5: Horny Goat Weed

Background: For several thousand years, Chinese medicine had administered horny goat weed, also known as *epimedium* or *yin yang huo*, as an aphrodisiac to increase libido. This leafy plant grows in the wild at high altitudes in China.

Findings: Horny goat weed extracts were used on rabbits and successfully relaxed the smooth muscle that corresponds to erectile pathways in men. The research team concluded that the herb is a possible treatment strategy for men with erectile dysfunction.[8]

Second study: A 2008 report by a team of researchers at the University of Milan (Italy), published in the *Journal of Natural Products*, found that a compound inside horny goat weed called icariin acts in the same way that Viagra's active compound, sildenafil, does to promote male erections. But whereas Viagra isn't recommended for people with heart problems, horny goat weed "appears to be safe," with no side effects, according to the researchers. The soft, green heart-shaped leaf of the horny goat weed "worked as well as Viagra" while causing "fewer side effects than Viagra," the study concludes.[9]

Study 6: BetterMAN

Background: BetterMAN is a product that blends eighteen traditional Chinese herbs, including ginseng root and horny goat weed.

Findings: A group of rats was fed this herbal mixture for two months, and their "erectile response was significantly better" than that of the control group of rats. "The mechanism of the herbal medicine is unknown," comment the study authors.[10]

Nature's Not-So-Secret Erectile Dysfunction Remedy

Another naturally occurring treatment for erectile dysfunction traditionally used in Asian cultures has received a seal of approval from numerous medical studies.

Korean red ginseng got its first major boost in 1995 when the *International Journal of Impotence Research* reported on a study in which ninety men with erectile dysfunction were divided into three groups: one group used Korean red ginseng, a second was given just a placebo, and the third got a pharmaceutical drug treatment. The ginseng group experienced "significantly higher" penile rigidity and girth and libido enhancement.[11]

More studies showing similar results followed. In 2002, for instance, the *Journal of Urology* published the results of a double-blind placebo-controlled study that found "significant improvement" in erectile function for Korean red ginseng users, which prompted the study authors to proclaim it "effective for treating male erectile dysfunction."[12]

A Synergistic Cure for Dysfunctions

One of the most rigorously studied natural dietary supplements for both male and female sexual dysfunctions is a product called ArginMax, distributed by the Daily Wellness Company, based in Mountain View, California. This product combines ginkgo biloba, Korean ginseng, the amino acid L-arginine, damiana, and twelve other vitamin and mineral ingredients into a proprietary formula that seems to work synergistically.

It was formulated by Dr. Hank Wuh, who got his MD from Johns Hopkins University Medical School and other degrees from Harvard University and Stanford University. Wuh's Chinese ancestry helped to inspire him to investigate the claims made for thousands of years by practitioners of Chinese traditional medicine that certain herbs have aphrodisiac properties.

At least four major medical studies published in prominent peer-reviewed journals (see page 142) have found this product to be beneficial for erectile dysfunction in men and for improving frequency of sexual desire, vaginal lubrication, and clitoral sensation in women. It may be the only product on the market with multiple ingredients that has yielded positive study results for both sexes. This should be especially heartening to women, because the pharmaceutical industry hasn't produced anything that works as a treatment for female sexual dysfunction.

An independent observer, neurophysiologist Beverly Whipple, a professor emerita at Rutgers University and president of the Society for the Scientific Study of Sexuality, had this to say about ArginMax in an interview with Salon.com: "I've been involved in research on women's sexuality for over 30 years. I was impressed by the ArginMax studies. The drug companies treat women as though they're mini-men. They can't understand why Viagra doesn't work for women. Well, it doesn't. But in a double-blind, placebo-controlled trial, ArginMax did. As a neurophysiologist, I find that very interesting. If women have problems with their sexual satisfaction, I think ArginMax is worth a try."[13]

Here is a summary of the four studies and their results:

1. In the *Journal of Sex & Marital Therapy*, a double-blind placebo-controlled study of seventy-seven women interested in improving their sexual function divided them into a placebo group and a group receiving ArginMax. After four weeks, 75.5 percent of the ArginMax group experienced greater satisfaction with their overall sex life, more sexual desire and clitoral sensation, and reduction of vaginal dryness. Only one-third of the placebo group reported any improvements. No significant side effects were found from use of the supplement.[14]

2. In the *Journal of Women's Health*, a study by researchers at Stanford University Medical School divided ninety-three women, ages twenty-two to seventy-three years, into placebo and ArginMax groups. After four weeks, those taking the supplement "reported significant improvements in level of sexual desire, satisfaction with sex life, and frequency of intercourse as compared to the placebo group. Significant improvements also were noted in lubrication, frequency of sexual desire, and degree of clitoral sensation."[15]

3. A 2006 study in the *Journal of Sex & Marital Therapy* worked with 108 women, twenty-two to seventy-three years old, who had reported a lack of sexual desire. They were divided into placebo and ArginMax groups. Once again, the women who took the supplement experienced significant improvement in their levels of sexual desire, their sexual satisfaction, and their clitoral sensitivity. "Since ArginMax for women has been shown to exhibit no estrogen activity," comment the study authors, "it may be a desirable alternative to hormone therapy for sexual concerns."[16]

4. Finally, in a study of men, a team of medical researchers based at the University of Hawaii School of Medicine did a four-week evaluation of seventy-three men, ages thirty-one to seventy-three years, who reported mild, moderate, or severe erectile dysfunction. By the end of the study, 87.5 percent of men in the ArginMax group had an improved ability

to maintain an erection, compared to just 22 percent in the placebo group. No side effects were reported from use of the supplement.[17]

Did You Know?

Aphrodisiacs Were Chosen by Shape

Ancient cultures selected their sex-enhancing potions based on two considerations: they ate fruits and plants that resembled human sexual organs, and they ate the genitals or bodily protrusions of powerful animals to acquire their attributes.

In the latter case, genitals and testicles from rams and bulls were prized. Elephant tusks, because they resembled erect penises, were pulverized into powder and consumed in Asia. Rhinoceros horns were exalted in Africa and Asia as virility boosters. Our term for sexual arousal, *horny*, comes from the belief that animal horns confer sexual vitality benefits.

For roots, fruits, and vegetables, the thinking among ancient cultures was that nature must have designed the shapes as a signpost indicating how they were to be used. So the ginseng root, for example, with its resemblance to a torso with arms and legs, became a symbol for sexual vitality. Bananas, cucumbers, carrots, and asparagus all became phallic symbols.

By luck, observation, intuition, or even the placebo effect, many of these reputed aphrodisiacs turned out to actually work in some people — ginseng being a good example — and their reputations grew.

In the case of the ancient cure-all ginkgo, a 1996 study in the *Journal of Urology* reported that ginkgo extracts can relax vascular smooth muscles in the penis to aid in the treatment of impotence.[18]

Beware of Fake "Natural" Aphrodisiacs

Numerous herbal sexual enhancement products marketed with the claim of containing "all-natural" ingredients have been exposed as containing the active ingredients in Viagra, Levitra, and Cialis without listing them. This consumer deception can endanger the health of anyone taking prescription nitrate drugs for diabetes, hypertension, or various other health problems. The active ingredients in prescription treatments for erectile dysfunction can interact with nitrates to cause a drastic and dangerous drop in the user's blood pressure.

A series of health alerts have been issued over the past few years to consumers by the U.S. Food and Drug Administration (FDA) based on its lab analyses of sexual enhancement supplements that were sold over the counter and on the Internet. Here are a few of the most notable cases from the FDA files:

2003: Manufacturers of Vinarol and Viga tablets, promoted as increasing desire, confidence, and sexual performance, issued recalls of those products when sildenafil, the active ingredient in Viagra, was found in both of them. That same year, manufacturers of Sigra, Stamina Rx, Stamina Rx for Women, Y-Y Spontane ES, and Uroprin were forced to recall those brands because they contained tadalafil, the active ingredient in Cialis.

2006: Manufacturers of Zimaxx, Libidus, Neophase, Nasutra, Vigor-25, Actra-Rx, and 4Everon were all cited by the FDA for marketing illegal drugs with the unlabeled and undeclared ingredients sildenafil or vardenafil, the active ingredient in Levitra.

2007: The manufacturer of Liviro3, Ebek, Inc., of Los Angeles, conducted a voluntary recall after an FDA lab analysis found tadalafil in its product. Later that year, Confidence, Inc., of Port Washington, New York, recalled its supplement Long Weekend, marketed under the American Best Nutrition label, after undeclared tadalafil was found to be an ingredient. Finally, Jen-On Herbal Science International of Industry, California, withdrew its HS Joy of Love product after vardenafil was found in it, and America True Man Health, Inc., of West Covina, California, was forced to recall its True Man Sexual Energy Nutrient Capsules and Energy Max Energy Supplement Men's Formula Capsules after sildenafil was found in them.

Some "Aphrodisiacs" Can Kill You

Toads are definitely not something you should kiss to improve your sex life.

A thirty-five-year-old man died in New York City in May 2008 after using the purported aphrodisiac toad venom, a hardened resin that comes mostly from China and is marketed under such names as Piedra, Love Stone, Jamaican Stone, or Chinese Rock.

His death came in the wake of five other deaths in New York involving users of the product, which is sold in neighborhood grocery stores and sex shops. "There is no safe way to use it," Dr. Robert Hoffman, director of New York's poison control center, told the news media. "Don't buy it. Don't use it. If you have it, throw it out!"[19]

Good Health Is the Best Aphrodisiac

Sexuality is the most interesting subject to everyone. Start a conversation about it and everyone stops and listens. It's the strongest motivation we have to live. But there are also absurdities when it comes to being sexually desirable. The true image of sexuality is vitality and health, not the marketing images created to sell products.

A study on sexuality in the journal *Sexual and Relationship Therapy* concludes that "sexual satisfaction is a major contributor to quality of life, ranking at least as highly as spiritual and religious commitments and other morale factors."[20]

People who like themselves generally feel sexier and more desirable to others. We are attracted to the vital and energetic person. The maintenance of good health probably has more to do with being sexually attractive than any other factor. Continued sexual activity and expression throughout life enhance the masculine feelings of men and the feminine feelings of women. Charisma probably is the hormonal connection we feel to a healthy and vital person.

Preserving passion in your life not only will prolong your life but will bless you with a more intense level of happiness and fulfillment than you would receive otherwise. Intensify your passion, and you intensify your enjoyment of life.

Ovulation Attracts Money from Men

Even though human females, unlike female animals, don't normally flaunt their ovulation, the intoxicating scent of fertility still attracts and affects the human male at his subconscious level of awareness.

To test that proposition, several University of New Mexico psychologists tracked the tips made by eighteen lap dancers over a two-month period at so-called gentlemen's clubs to see if ovulation cycles made a difference in the amount of money the women made rubbing themselves against male customers.

During their peak of fertility, the dancers made an average of seventy dollars an hour, compared to just thirty-five dollars while menstruating and fifty dollars when between cycles.

"These results have clear implications for human evolution, sexuality, and economics," conclude the study authors.[21]

One cannot help but wonder if women throughout history haven't intuitively known this all along.

Techniques to Jump-Start Your Libido

Beds have been called the best piece of fitness equipment that you can buy. But you don't always need to be bouncing on one to improve your sexual performance.

Pelvic floor exercises can restore erectile function in many men who suffer from an inability to achieve and maintain an erection.

This no-cost natural alternative to Viagra was thoroughly examined in a 2005 British experiment that worked with fifty-five men afflicted by erectile dysfunction. They were divided into two groups. One group received instruction from a physiotherapist on pelvic floor muscle exercises they could perform at home, while the other group undertook no exercises and received only advice about changes in lifestyle that might improve their condition.

During their training, the exercise group was taught how to tighten their pelvic muscles as firmly as possible to build muscle strength. Special training attention was placed on developing the ability to retract the penis and lift the scrotum. Twice daily, participants did a series of these contractions while lying down, while sitting, and then while standing up. They were taught how to stop and start the flow of urine to further strengthen the muscles involved in erections.

After six months of these exercises, the results were both conclusive and startling. As the five authors of this study observe in the September 2005 issue of the *British Journal of Urology*, at least 40 percent of the men in the exercise group regained full normal erectile function, 35.5 percent improved their function, and only 24.5 percent showed no improvement. Some men also reported the return of erections in their sleep and on waking. Little improvement in erectile function occurred among men in the lifestyle changes–only group.

"In conclusion," write the study authors, "pelvic floor muscle exercises should be considered as a first-line approach for men seeking long-term resolution of erectile dysfunction without acute pharmacological and surgical interventions that might have more significant side-effects. Men demanding a 'quick fix' or a 'pill for every ill' might prefer to restore normal muscle function once they understand the important role of the pelvic floor muscles."[22]

Exercise in general remains the safest miracle tonic — next to dietary nutrients — for maintenance of sexual health. "Moderate regular exercise will help to improve blood flow to the sexual organs. In addition, exercise helps you feel good about yourself. Anything that improves self-esteem will improve libido," says Dr. Catherine Hood of Oxford University in England.[23]

You must exercise aerobically nearly every day, which will get blood to your genitalia. Weightlifting is also helpful. Certain leg-lift exercises and core building will bring more hormones into the genital area and enhance sexual desire.

In the aftermath of childbirth, the vaginal muscles in most women become flaccid, and without proper exercise attention, this flaccidity can result in decreased sensation and pleasure during intercourse for both partners. Various exercises can counteract this effect.

Also keep in mind that intercourse burns about 150 calories per half hour, compared to 129 calories per half hour spent dancing, 152 calories walking moderately fast, and 114 calories doing yoga. So sexual activity is an exercise that can help you lose weight if you engage in it with regularity.

The synergy of diet plus exercise can extend your life and improve and revitalize your sex life. That is the bottom-line message of this book.

Eight Ways to Keep Sex Interesting

1. **Plan for spontaneity.** This might sound like a contradiction in terms, but don't underestimate the power of scheduling your sexual encounters, yet leaving the details of what you intend to do open and subject to your spontaneous passion and combined imaginations. While single, you may have called these encounters a date, which is a ritual worth practicing even when you're married.

2. **Create adventures.** Doing new things together that you find exciting can stimulate deeper levels of bonding that can lead to a more exciting sex life. You don't have to jump out of airplanes together, though that might be worth trying, and you don't have to visit nude beaches, though that might be fun, too. You could learn ballroom dancing or even how to tango together. Just do something outside of your routine to help bring you closer together.

3. **Make foreplay more promiscuous.** Real foreplay isn't just about preparing each other for the sexual act. It's about building up desire over time, touch by touch. Show your affection toward each other in your everyday contact. A touch on the neck, a light kiss on the hand or forehead, a suggestive look or wink, even something as simple as making dinner together can all amp up the sexual voltage.

4. **Use "oral" sex with each other.** We all know what oral sex is,

or at least we think that we do. But before you actually go down on each other, try talking and listening to each other with a new level of intimacy. Share your fantasies, however forbidden they might feel. An intimate dialogue can be just as sexy as the act itself because your imagination is doing the lovemaking.

5. Develop sensual rituals. To transition between our normal routines and our professional and family roles in life, we need rituals that can bring us through the door of intimacy. Sharing a shower together is one tension breaker. Giving each other a massage can be another. Even reading to each other, especially if it's sensual or sexually provocative literature, can help you bridge the gap between feeling obligations and expressing intimacy.

6. Keep pride in your appearance. You probably know how easy it is to let the little things slide and for complacency to set in. He forgets to shave or no longer thinks that it's important. She thinks wearing jeans or a sweatshirt all the time is okay. Even basic hygiene can sometimes go by the wayside in long-term relationships. Never take your appearance for granted! To be sexy and to feel sexy, you always need pride in how you look.

7. Go somewhere new. We all know how vacations sometimes bring out desires and feelings that were wilting away in the background of our lives. Take short trips, a night or a weekend, and go somewhere new and stimulating to break the routine. Variety is indeed the spice of life, and the more you experiment with new settings, the fresher your sexual connection can feel.

8. Don't forget fantasy. The most powerful aphrodisiac is found in our imaginations, and we should use that tool for sexual intimacy whenever we can. Try playing different roles with each other. You could even go to a restaurant and pretend that you don't know each other. Try to pick each other up using

a different persona. By acting out these roles, you might discover some new and exciting aspect of yourself or your partner.

Qigong Your Sex Drive

Historians tell us that Chinese emperors, thousands of years ago, kept hundreds of young concubines to satisfy their sexual desires. Some of these emperors lived into their seventies or eighties, yet Chinese chroniclers claimed they remained sexually active with multiple members of their harems.

If these accounts are correct, a clue to their sexual prowess might be found in an ancient Chinese practice called Qigong (pronounced "chi-kung") that uses a combination of body postures, controlled breathing exercises, and visualizations for health and healing. Practitioners of Qigong believe that it also offers the promise of supercharging your sex drive and enhancing your level of sexual pleasure and expression. They claim it can heal sexual dysfunctions, relieve PMS symptoms in women, stimulate whole-body orgasms, and even channel sexual energy toward creating better overall physical health.

Some of the exercises associated with sexual Qigong involve shaking and vibrating the sex organs, along with holding and massaging the organs and surrounding areas to "charge" them. Visualizations are intended to focus the mind on sex and the sex organs to accompany and facilitate body movements. These exercises can be done in sitting, standing, and sleeping positions. (To learn a few of these exercises, access www.super qigong.com/articlesmore.asp?id=84.)

Basic Qigong movement and meditation exercises can be found in numerous videos and books that have been produced on the subject. Most practitioners advise that the exercises be taught by trained instructors, many of whom are associated with martial arts schools. Check out the Internet for Qigong classes and instructors near you — there are many schools and traditions to choose among — and inquire about whether they specialize in the sexual toning afforded by the practice. This practice is an important part of the Hippocrates program.

Dozens of books about Qigong are available, with two popular ones being *The Essential Qigong Training Course* and *The Way of Qigong*, both by Ken Cohen.

Prolong Your Sexuality

*Sexual intercourse is
kicking death in the ass while singing.*

—Novelist Charles Bukowski (1920–1994)

There Is No Age Limit to Good Sex

*Is it not strange that desire
should so many years outlive performance?*

— Playwright William Shakespeare (1564–1616)

Alicia and her husband, Charles, are one of the more delightful and en-
ergetically happy couples we have ever known. They have been married
for sixty years and show no evidence of having diminished their love and
passion for each other. They fall asleep holding hands every night, and in
the morning they always kiss each other to start their day. "We've made
love thousands of times," says Charles, "and the last time is always the
lovemaking we remember as being the best."

Alicia overcame cancer in the 1990s, but the disease was just a speed
bump on their road of life. They have remained youthful in appearance,

health, and spirit by eating a pure whole-foods diet and by treating each new day as an opportunity for learning and adventure. It all began in Massachusetts on their second date in 1948, when Charles took Alicia up in a stunt plane and did a series of loops and spins. Though Alicia promptly threw up her last meal, a tradition was established between them: nothing in their lives together was going to be boring.

Much later in life, they made love in the bathroom of a 747 airliner on the way to Australia. For his eightieth birthday, Alicia took Charles on a nudist cruise in the Caribbean with several thousand other nudists, sponsored by the cruise company Bare Necessities. But the sexual exercise they've most enjoyed in their eighties has been ballroom dancing. "The intimacy of ballroom dancing, the touching, the movement, the eye contact, it's all good foreplay," says Alicia. "Saturdays are set aside as our intimacy and lovemaking days. Love, rather than animal instinct, is the sexual stimulant for us. The years have brought us more romance, and there's no better aphrodisiac than good health and a good partner."

We had another guest at Hippocrates named Margaret, ninety-three years old, an energetic and bright-eyed great-grandmother, who told us that she still has desire for men. She talks about chasing after younger men in their seventies because "the old farts my age aren't worth anything in bed." She isn't in fantasyland concerning her interest in sex. Her attitude is healthy, even if it is rare. She perceives herself as still being attractive to the opposite sex, regardless of her age or theirs. When we abandon desire and being desirable, we begin to give up on life. But if we retain and cultivate desire, it helps us to remain vital, and Margaret is a living example and testament to that.

Guests at Hippocrates undergo major vitality improvements while they are experiencing our program. We don't know of anyone who has maintained the dietary lifestyle that we teach here who hasn't experienced a better sex life and a stronger level of desire. We hear that from guests all the time. Elderly people who maintain our diet make love a lot more often than many of the young people we see who have unhealthy dietary and lifestyle habits.

This doesn't conflict with the fact that aging can have an effect on sexuality. Aging's impact on sexual functioning has been well documented in the medical literature. For men, testosterone levels decline with age until their sexual response cycle resembles that of a woman — they have a greater need for longer periods spent in foreplay and more tactile stimulation to achieve erection and climax. Estrogen levels rise as men get older, giving them more feminine characteristics that include breast growth. The failure of some men to understand and accept these natural bodily and sexual changes can result in anxiety, depression, and a continuing cycle of dysfunction.

For women, natural hormone levels decline, as does the sharpness of their olfactory functioning. Smell is most associated with sexual stimulation in women, more so than in men, because this sense regulates their emotional states. All these symptoms of aging, combined with unavailability of sexual partners in their own age group, can diminish the intensity of sexual desire that many women feel late in life. But it would be a mistake to think these are the primary reasons that many members of both sexes forsake their sexuality in their autumn years.

At a certain point in the later stages of their lives, many men and women simply abandon, with reluctance and regret, any interest in expressing their sexuality. The reasons for this abandonment often have little or no relationship to their true desires and wishes, but are a result of lowered expectations engineered by a loss of hope.

A British survey of sexual activity and attitudes among the elderly, published in a 2003 issue of *Social Science and Medicine*, underscores the toxic impact of judgments and attitudes, finding that "participants who did not consider sex to be of any importance to them neither had a current sexual partner, nor felt that they would have another sexual partner in their lifetime. Indeed, all participants who had a current sexual partner attributed at least some importance to sex, with many rating sex as 'very' or 'extremely' important. However, experiencing barriers to being sexually active led them to place less importance on sex."[1]

One big psychological barrier frequently imposed on elders' sexual expression is the judgment of younger relatives or caregivers that sex among the elderly is "repugnant," "dangerous," or even "morally wrong." As an article in a 2005 issue of the *Journal of Sex Research* pointed out, "Attitudes are more significant influences on sexual desire than bio-medical factors," which include hormone levels, illness, and the effects of medications on libido.[2]

In a 1977 study of forty nursing home staffers, a prevailing belief was found that sexual activity among older people must be less moral or less important than sex among younger people. This turns out to be a common ageist stereotype among nursing home personnel, and it works to discourage sexual activity by the elderly in numerous ways, including the creation of barriers to privacy.[3] To illustrate how prevalent this has become, a 1979 survey of sixty-three nursing home residents found that 81 percent of the men and 75 percent of the women admitted to having sexual thoughts and fantasies, yet few acted on their urges because of a lack of opportunity. The study authors conclude that a lack of privacy in nursing homes is a major obstacle to sexual expression.[4]

By welcome contrast, a 1985 survey of 140 medical students indicated that most viewed sexually active older people as being significantly more mentally alert, cheerful, and better adjusted.[5] So while the negative impact of judgments and attitudes on sexual behaviors in a caregiver environment cannot be overstated, neither should we overlook, nor undervalue, the health benefits of positive sexual activity. If nursing home personnel and other caregivers are truly concerned with the mental and physical health of their clients, they will begin to loosen the constraints that inhibit healthy sexual expression.

Young women are sexualized and sexually objectified in our culture, while older women are considered to be neither sexual nor sexually attractive beings. Such societal attitudes and beliefs can become a self-fulfilling prophecy when older men and women begin to conform their sexual thoughts, activities, and sexual relationships to these ageist conceits and prejudices. "Physiological changes in sexual function (based on aging) can affect libido and performance, but these effects have been overestimated relative to those caused by psychological and emotional issues," emphasized a 2002 study in the journal *Sexual and Relationship Therapy*.[6]

We have a lithe, physically fit, and very vital associate working with us at Hippocrates who is seventy-two years old, but if you saw her, you'd think she was twenty years younger. Lizanne grew up in Cleveland, Ohio, and lived a rather traditional married life, birthing five children by the time she was twenty-seven; then the sexual revolution of the '60s swept her up in its riptide, and she abandoned her marriage for sexual experimentation. "I learned that free love was a lousy idea for me," she says today. "It was empty and unfulfilling."

Lizanne makes some important points about sex and aging — "If you keep exercising and eat healthy, your libido should remain intact" — and about the cultural stereotypes that continue to discourage women past the age of sixty from seeing themselves as desirable sexual beings. "The media has a lot to do with the image that older people aren't sexual. Movies usually portray older people, especially women, as surrounded by bottles of pills and walkers and wheelchairs, and languishing in nursing homes. The actor and sex symbol Sean Connery is my age, but he's always paired in movies with young women in their twenties and thirties. When are we going to see women my age paired in movies with handsome men thirty or forty years younger?"

After counseling literally thousands of people, we found the overwhelming majority, no matter what age they are, still have a desire to remain sexually active. Several times a week we meet people in their seventies, eighties, or even nineties who ask us, "How can we become virile again? How can we find our libidos again?" The stigma on the aged population going back to Puritan times (not that we aren't in Puritan times still) is branded on our cultural consciousness.

Some people think it's almost abnormal to have sexual relationships past a certain age. We strongly disagree. There is no one who is healthy in their mind who doesn't still have a desire for sexual intimacy. One of the great reasons for living to old age is to continue sharing that intimacy.

A couple of generations ago, when one lost a spouse, it was almost a mortal sin to be intimate with someone afterward. One either continued wearing black to symbolize mourning, or put a dark veil over one's spirit. Today, thankfully, this cultural proscription has changed. People lose one or even two spouses and take on another. That's healthy because it shows your biological clock is still ticking. It keeps us alive and vital.

Common Myths about Aging and Sexuality

Assisted living should bring an end to sexuality: It's true that far too many nursing homes and assisted living facilities are sterile environments. You're supposed to behave, which means the sexes are separated and no one is supposed to have sex or intimacy. I (Anna Maria) worked in a private nursing home and saw this situation firsthand. It's not an environment designed for intimacy. It's a warehouse where sex as a natural need is shunned and forgotten. It doesn't have to be this way! Institutional attitudes need to change.

Aging may sometimes limit, but it need never eliminate, sexual performance for men or women. In fact, many couples develop new sexual skills late in life, owing in part to heightened patience and an ability to laugh and not take sex so seriously.

Women don't have as much sexual desire as men: This is more cultural conditioning. Women don't peak sexually until their thirties and forties; look at the trend of older women marrying much younger men. That's a reflection, in part, of their sexual desire levels. We've talked to hundreds of women who say sex is more satisfying after menopause, partly because the concern about pregnancy is gone. (It's important for women to keep in mind that vaginal dryness isn't a universal condition and that it is a correctable one.)

You can't be sexy after a certain age: This is a common myth and perhaps the most enduring one in western cultures. While they may not have the hard bodies of twenty-year-olds, mature women can still be very sexy. It really comes down to exercise, proper diet, and good grooming and hygiene. Though the media may attempt to condition and teach us that when we reach a certain age we should hold a low opinion of our bodies and our sexuality, it's really nonsense and silly to think sex can't be exciting at seventy or eighty years of age.

Infamous Sex Myth

Sex Increases Men's Stroke and Heart Attack Risk

In the early 1980s, a fear arose among many men and women that sexual activity could increase a man's risk of stroke and heart attack. This heightened concern came in the aftermath of former U.S. Vice President Nelson Rockefeller's well-publicized death from a heart attack while engaged in sexual intercourse with a woman who was not his wife.

Subsequent medical studies should have put most of those concerns to rest. For example, a 2002 study in the *Journal of Epidemiology and Community Health*, by a team of British medical researchers, surveyed 914 men (aged forty-five to fifty-nine years) during the period 1979 to 1983, then surveyed them again twenty years later.

Their conclusion: "Middle-aged men should be heartened to know that frequent sexual intercourse is not likely to result in a substantial increase in risk of strokes, and that some protection from fatal coronary events may be an added bonus."[7]

Infamous Sex Myth

Menopause Means the End of Sexual Desire

How many times have you heard someone say about a woman entering menopause, "There goes her sex drive"? Or maybe you've even had this thought about yourself based on how postmenopausal women have described their lives.

Medical science has demonstrated that this common perception that menopause equals the loss of desire is a myth. "The mature or postmenopausal woman need not abandon sexual intimacy," reads a 1998 report in the *Journal of Women's Health*. "Given the benefit of good health, a loving relationship, and appropriate medical care, sexual vigor can continue in the mature years of a woman's life."[8]

A 2004 study in the journal *Menopause* reached a similar conclusion: There is growing evidence against a "simple model of midlife sexuality that depicts women as victims of their bodily and hormonal changes. Instead, life stressors, contextual factors, past sexuality, and mental health problems are more significant predictors of midlife women's sexual interest than menopause status itself."[9]

Benefits of Natural Hormone Replacement Therapy

Endocrinologist Dr. Edward L. Klaiber, in his 2002 book *Hormones and the Mind*, emphasizes the importance of testosterone to a woman's sexual satisfaction — "Testosterone feeds the sexual mind," he writes — and summarizes the symptoms of hormone deficiencies in women this way: "For women at midlife, the sexual symptoms of estrogen deficiency are vaginal dryness and a thinning of the vaginal wall that make sexual relations more difficult and less satisfying. By contrast, the sexual symptoms of testosterone deficiency have been less publicized, but they are more encompassing. These symptoms include the diminution of sexual energy, drive, vitality, and orgasmic function."[10]

Natural testosterone, sometimes called the "hormone of desire," given its powerful effect on libido, given to women at one-tenth the dose used in men, can improve their sexual desire and responsiveness. Here are the six indicators of testosterone deficiency in women, as related by Dr. Susan Rako in her book *The Hormone of Desire*:

1. Decreased sexual desire, including a loss of desire to masturbate.
2. Diminished overall vital energy.
3. Less sensitivity to sexual stimulation in the clitoris.
4. Less sensitivity to sexual stimulation in the nipples.
5. Decreased arousability and orgasm capacity.
6. Thinning of the pubic hair.[11]

A loss of interest in sex, thinning hair, weight gain, and lethargy are all symptoms many people chalk up to normal aging. Bioidentical hormone replacement therapy has emerged to alleviate these symptoms. These hormones are molecularly identical to the hormones produced in the body, whose production is diminished by aging.

Several synthetic hormone replacement drugs manufactured from animal waste have been linked in medical studies to raising women's risk of stroke, heart attack, and breast cancer. By contrast, natural bioidentical hormones are taken from plants, especially wild yams, and are applied as creams directly to the skin to avoid problems associated with the oral delivery of synthetics.

DHEA is a testosterone precursor harvested in a natural way from wild yams. The best source of DHEA is a liquid wild yam extract. Several companies worldwide sell it. Synthetic laboratory DHEA doesn't have the cofactors or the subcultures that allow it to develop the body hormones necessary for proper functioning.

Though natural hormone replacement therapy was developed primarily for women, men can also benefit from it. Aging men go through hormonal changes (often called male menopause) that include a loss of testosterone, which results in loss of sexual interest, impotence, thinning hair, diminished physical endurance, and even depression. Testosterone replacement can alleviate these symptoms.

A simple saliva test, similar to a blood test, can measure the specific levels of hormones that are missing in the body. Based on these results, physicians can prescribe precise dosages of bioidentical DHEA, estrogen, testosterone, and progesterone. Unlike prescription synthetics, these natural doses can be tailored to the individual needs of each person for optimal benefit to health and sexual fulfillment.

Male Menopause Isn't a Myth

At a certain stage of middle age, some men report many of the symptoms common to women who are experiencing menopause. These symptoms in men, according to the Mayo Clinic, can include the following:

- hot flushes and sweats
- reduced sexual desire
- swollen and tender breasts
- loss of body and pubic hair
- feeling sad or depressed
- sleep problems
- poor concentration or memory
- decreased energy[12]

First reported in the medical literature in 1944, male menopause might more accurately be called *andropause*, which means a decrease in testosterone levels. Unlike menopause in women, which is marked by a defined age range in which hormone production stops, male andropause can be a slow but steady decline over many years. It has also been called "irritable male syndrome."

A January 2004 article in the *New England Journal of Medicine* reported low testosterone in 9 percent of men in their forties, 30 percent of men in their fifties, 42 percent of men in their sixties, and 70 percent or more of men in their seventies. Other studies have shown that men with low testosterone levels don't live as long as men with "normal" levels.[13]

Physical effects of low testosterone can include osteoporosis, pre-diabetes and diabetes, increased body fat linked to heart disease, abnormal blood fat, and increased risk for atherosclerosis. "It is time for men (and their spouses, partners and physicians) to become aware that testosterone in men is not just a sex hormone but a total body hormone, essential for normal psychological and physical functioning and to help offset risks for chronic life-threatening diseases," says Dr. Harvey S. Bartnof, director of the California Longevity & Vitality Medical Institute in San Francisco.[14]

Male menopause can be alleviated to some extent by regular exercise, a healthy diet, and other lifestyle changes. It should also be noted that a male midlife crisis may sometimes resemble andropause due to depression and related problems that arise when males confront their loss of vitality and youth.

Sexual Expression Lengthens Life Spans

Sexuality is a deep, rich well that older couples gain strength from when health crises occur. As noted earlier, it wasn't too many years ago that when someone lost a spouse at an early age, they would remain widows or widowers for the rest of their lives.

It isn't the intent of nature that your life should end when you lose your partner. Nor is it the intent of nature that your sexuality should end when you lose your mate. That would be suppression of the human spirit. In some cultures, widows wore black as a sign of mourning until they died. Today, finding a second partner after the loss of the first is common. Why should anyone accept loneliness or think it's a normal circumstance?

Some people have been so hurt by sexual relationships that they say they'd rather be alone, as if that were somehow normal. But no matter what they say, no one would rather be alone. Everyone wants a partner and the happiness that can potentially develop over time from a caring relationship.

We all need to be nourished sexually. While it's normal to have lower levels of sex hormones as we age, if we stay sexually active, we spawn a higher level of these necessary hormones. Being in a committed relationship increases your chances of keeping those hormone levels higher than would be the case if you were alone.

Abandoning sexual desire takes away the greatest overriding reason that you are alive: to propagate our species. Even when you are past your fertile years, though, sexual desire remains, like a drum that never stops beating, even though you may stop listening.

According to all the available medical evidence, intimacy and marriage can produce great and powerful long-term benefits. "At older ages, married men and women face lower risks of sexual dysfunction than the unmarried of the same age," reports the International Longevity Center. "Being married has been shown to have consistently positive effects on health and longevity."[15]

Never lose sight of the fact that sex can be a kind of Fountain of Youth. "Sexuality is a life-giving energy that holds back the curtain of death" is the apt way that Annie Laura Cotten, an emeritus professor of psychology at Central Connecticut State University, describes it.[16]

Major Scientific Studies Support Our Viewpoint

Medical science has uncovered a lot of evidence to support what we contend in this book to be true about the link between sexuality and aging:

- Orgasm frequency extends life and "may be protective of middle-aged men's health." Mortality risk was 50 percent lower in men with high orgasmic frequency, found a study of 918 men in Wales.[17]
- In a study of 2,453 elderly women and men in Taiwan, it was shown that the absence of libido and lessened sexual activity produced a much higher mortality rate in comparison to those elderly who continued having sexual relations.[18]
- A study of 3,500 people up to the age of 101 found that regular sexual activity "helps you to look four to seven years younger," based on impartial photo ratings and analysis.[19]
- The quality and frequency of sexual expression in older adults "is itself a predictor of good general health and well-being."[20]
- Having a sexual partner in old age contributes toward good mental health, and that is particularly true in older women who are threatened by ill health.[21]

Age Is Mostly Just a State of Mind

In a study of nursing homes, Harvard University professor of psychology Ellen J. Langer, PhD, comes to this conclusion about the impact of attitudes on aging: "The notion that the aging process and the physical deterioration that accompanies it are the inevitable results of the passage of time sets us up for a self-fulfilling prophecy."[22]

To underscore this view, Professor Langer and some Harvard graduate students undertook a fascinating experiment in the 1980s to test attitudes and their impact on aging. They recruited a group of men ages seventy-five to eighty, and tested what would happen if they adopted states of mind they had had at fifty-five years of age.

The male volunteers were divided into two groups: an experimental group and a control group. All the volunteers were brought together at a retreat facility and weren't allowed access to any books, newspapers, magazines, or family photos that were less than two decades old. Throughout the experiment, members of each group were tested for physical strength, perception, cognition, taste, hearing, and vision.

The experimental group made a psychological attempt to "be the person they were" twenty years earlier. They engaged in present-time conversations with one another, as if they were truly reliving the way they had been two decades earlier. They were given photos of one another from decades earlier and were encouraged to actually return their minds to that earlier period in their lives and let themselves be who they were in 1959. To reinforce that state of mind, this group was exposed only to *Life* and *Saturday Evening Post* magazines and radio and television programs from 1959. They viewed movies from that era and had conversations about sports teams as if those teams and their stars still played.

By contrast, the control group conversed about themselves only in the past tense, simply retrieving memories about their lives in 1959. They were only given photos of one another that were recent. They also had access to periodicals and radio and television programs since the 1959 period.

Differences between the two groups after a week ranged from "the striking to the suggestive," Langer writes. Joint flexibility "increased to a significantly greater degree" in the experimental group, with their finger length actually increasing by over a third; their sitting height also increased. By contrast, the control group members experienced a worsening of flexibility. The experimental group members also gained strength and dexterity, improved their eyesight, and had improved intelligence test scores. The control group showed none of these improvements.

So-called irreversible signs of aging were reversed in the experimental group using this mindfulness intervention. That led Professor Langer to conclude, "The regular and 'irreversible' cycles of aging that we witness in the later stages of human life may be a product of certain assumptions about how one is supposed to grow old. If we didn't feel compelled to carry out these limiting mind-sets, we might have a greater chance of replacing years of decline with years of growth and purpose."[23]

Join the Boomer Sexual Liberation Front

Maybe you saw the headlines when they appeared in November 2010: "Baby Boomers Unhappy with Their Sex Lives, Study Finds."

Here is how that Associated Press story began: "The generation that promoted free love has grown old and cranky about sex. Faced with performance problems, menopause blues and an increased mismatch of expectations between the sexes, baby boomers are the unhappiest Americans of all when it comes to making love."[24]

This conclusion was based on interviews across the United States with 945 people ages forty-five to sixty-five, followed by interviews with an additional 587 people ages eighteen to forty-four, and over sixty-five. Among boomers, 24 percent expressed dissatisfaction with their sex lives, compared to just 12 percent of the younger people and only 17 percent of those over sixty-five.

How did this boomer dissatisfaction happen?

The boomer generation, born between the years 1946 and 1964, had been at the forefront of the revolution in sexual attitudes and sexual experimentation that started in the "free love" 1960s. Whatever you might think of the '60s — that it was a refreshing and liberating era or a decadent and overly permissive period — it's undeniable that the people who lived through it transformed our sexual landscape forever and in a myriad of ways.

Take those lyrics from the Crosby, Stills, Nash and Young song "Love the One You're With." Until the 1960s, the socially acceptable thing to do if your spouse died was to remain single and celibate until you died, too. That attitude changed. We began to understand that you don't have to love just one person for your entire life, unless you choose to. We're capable of loving many people.

The sexual revolution liberated us from the dark cloud over sexual expression that our parents inherited. We're still a rebellious generation. We aren't going quietly to the grave. We aren't going to act old in our seventies and beyond. We're going to defy the social norms and expectations about what aging should look like and feel like.

So how do we account for the study results? It comes back to the word *expectations*. Too many boomers held on to the unrealistic expectation that their sex lives would just naturally remain wild and exciting and at peak performance levels throughout their days, without ever taking into account what poor nutrition and lack of proper exercise do to the sex drive and sexual performance. Good sex later in life requires some thought, discipline, and hard work, all of which boomers are capable of if they put their idealism and energies toward the task.

Becoming older shouldn't be seen as an ordeal to be endured. Boomers need to be leading the way in developing sex-positive approaches to aging and health. Some are already at the forefront of this new awareness. Many boomers are rejecting the idea that the aging process should discourage them from pursuing an active and passionate life right up until death, which means remaining vigorously active. So why not reject the idea that sex has to be boring or predictable?

In our experience, we find many exceptions to the study findings. Fred, forty-eight years old, a registered dietician who has been married for a decade, provides a typical boomer case. This native New Yorker describes for us how he and his wife are "at the highest peak of our sexual energy flow right now, better than ever before," thanks in large measure to a more wholesome diet. "We can never see ourselves not having sex in our later years. Our interests might change, the frequency might change, but we can't imagine our desire for each other will diminish. We both feel that sex in old age is essential to good health."

Boomers can set an intention to age gracefully, or at least to not look or act old. Just as many boomers will never willingly go into retirement, they should not give up on cultivating a memorable sex life. As our culture's attitudes about aging and sexuality change, so will its attitudes about the role of senior citizens as healthy and productive role models.

We had all sorts of "liberation" fronts in the '60s. Now it's time for a new one — the Boomer Sexual Liberation Front. Let our generation lead the way to healthier sex, less guilt and shame, and much longer, more fulfilling lives.

Resources

Websites about Sacred Sexuality

Tantra.com: This website is devoted to sacred sexuality and features instructional videos and books for those seeking a spiritual approach to sex. Articles can be found here on ejaculation control for men, how to be multiorgasmic, tantric massage, and female ejaculation. A tantra teacher directory gives listings of instructors near you who give personalized lessons or group tantra workshops.

BarbaraCarrellas.com: She is a sex educator who authored *Urban Tantra: Sacred Sex for the Twenty-First Century* and promotes conscious sexuality based on sacred practices such as tantra.

TheShameFreeZone.com: Maintained by sexologist Veronica Monet, based in Northern California, this website features a variety of useful information about relationships and sex, emphasizing sex-positive advice.

YourSexCoach.com: Sexologist Dr. Patti Britton, author of *The Idiot's Guide to Sensual Massage* and the audiobook *Sex: Tantra & Kama Sutra*, maintains this website devoted to healthy expressions of sexuality.

Sex-Positive Organizations and Treatment Centers

AASECT.org: This is the home site of the American Association of Sexuality Educators, Counselors and Therapists, which maintains listings of certified sex therapists throughout the United States.

SexHelp.com: This site was created by sex addictions expert Dr. Patrick Carnes and hosts a sex questionnaire that could be helpful in determining whether you have a sex compulsion problem.

Sex-Positive Marital Aids

Adult Movies and Books

Candida Royalle Productions: This former adult film star turned sex advice columnist pioneered the production of erotic films with a woman's perspective. Femme Productions was created in 1984 to produce adult films for couples that portray female concerns and desires in a healthy, sex-positive way. Candida authored a book, *How to Tell a Naked Man What to Do*, in which she explores how women can best understand their own sexual needs and desires, and then how to go about having those needs and desires met. She has since launched a new line of films called Femme Chocolat, featuring actresses and directors who are women of color (www.candidaroyalle.com).

AnnieSprinkle.org: Another adult film star who created her own line of instructional videos, such as *Amazing World of Orgasm*, in which twenty-six orgasm experts share their expertise on giving and receiving orgasms.

BettyDodson.com: Often called "the mother of female masturbation," this PhD sexologist and author of such books as *Sex for One* and *Orgasms for Two* offers instructional videos and a complete line of sex toys. Her website features advice columns and forums about sexuality, censorship, and other topics.

PuckerUp.com: Tristan Taormino is a sex educator, activist lesbian, and author of *The Ultimate Guide to Anal Sex for Women*, as well as the creator of instructional videos on anal sex and other subjects.

BetterSex.com: A site that offers a wide range of products from instructional videos and *The Better Sex* series (dealing with such topics as oral and anal sex) to adult sex toys and adult movies.

Notes

Foreword

1   See Bradley J. Willcox, D. Craig Willcox, and Makoto Suzuki, *The Okinawa Program: How the World's Longest-Lived People Achieve Everlasting Health — and How You Can Too* (New York: Three Rivers Press, 2002).

Introduction

Epigraph: John Callahan compiled the epigraphs for this book; see www.searchquotes.com (accessed November 1, 2011).

1   Ilya Petrou, "Global Better Sex Survey," *Urology Times*, June 2007, www.urologytimes.modernmedicine.com.

2   Bruce Lipton, *The Biology of Belief* (Carlsbad, CA: Hay House, 2005); Candace Pert, *Molecules of Emotion* (New York: Simon & Schuster, 1999).

Key One: Understand Your Sexuality

Epigraphs: Matt Groening, www.searchquotes.com (accessed November 1, 2011); Jane Austen, *Jane Austen: The Complete Novels* (London: Shoes and Ships and Sealing Wax, 2006), 460; Aldous Huxley, *Eyeless in Gaza* (New York: Harper & Brothers, 1936), ch. 27.

1   Charles Q. Choi, "Forecast: Sex and Marriage with Robots by 2050," *LiveScience*, October 12, 2007, www.livescience.com/1951-forecast-sex-marriage-robots-2050.html (accessed February 13, 2012).

2   Judith MacKay, "Global Sex: Sexuality and Sexual Practices around the World," *Sexual and Relationship Therapy* 16, no. 1 (2001): 71–82.

3 Simon LeVay, *The Sexual Brain* (Cambridge, MA: MIT Press, 1994), 137.

4 MacKay, "Global Sex," 74–77.

5 Lawrence B. Finer, "Trends in Premarital Sex in the United States, 1954–2003," *Public Health Reports* 122, no. 1 (January–February 2007): 73–78.

6 Emily Driscoll, "Bisexual Species," *Scientific American Mind* (June/July 2008): 68–73.

7 International Longevity Center, *Ageism in America* (New York: International Longevity Center, 2005–06), www.mailman.columbia.edu/academic-departments/centers/international-longevity-center/publications.

8 J. Mulhall et al., "Importance of and Satisfaction with Sex among Men and Women Worldwide: Results of the Global Better Sex Survey," *Journal of Sexual Medicine* 5, no. 4 (April 2008): 788–95; H. M. Tan et al., "Sex among Asian Men and Women: The Global Better Sex Survey in Asia," *International Journal of Urology* 16, no. 5 (May 2009): 507–15.

9 S. K. Fugl-Meyer et al., "On Orgasm, Sexual Techniques, and Erotic Perceptions in 18- to 74-Year-Old Swedish Women," *Journal of Sexual Medicine* 3, no. 1 (January 2006): 56–68.

10 International Longevity Center, *Ageism in America*.

11 Psychotherapist Donald Altman, MA, LPC, an expert on CBT, assisted with the preparation of the material on CBT. See www.mindfulpractices.com.

Key Two: Imagine Your Sexuality

1 Barnaby Barratt quoted in Dulce Zamora, "Good Food for Better Sex?," MedicineNet.com, www.medicinenet.com/script/main/art.sp?articlekey=56672 (accessed November 2, 2011).

2 Martin Portner, "The Orgasmic Mind," *Scientific American Mind* (April–May 2008): 67.

3 James Simon et al., "Testosterone Patch Increases Sexual Activity and Desire in Surgically Menopausal Women with Hypoactive Sexual Desire Disorder," *Journal of Clinical Endocrinology & Metabolism* 90, no. 9 (September 2005): 5226–33.

4 Jan L. Shifren et al., "Transdermal Testosterone Treatment in Women with Impaired Sexual Function after Oophorectomy," *New England Journal of Medicine* 343, no. 10 (September 7, 2000): 687.

5 Alfred Kinsey, *Sexual Behavior in the Human Female* (Philadelphia: W. B. Saunders, 1953).

6 Simon LeVay, *The Sexual Brain* (Cambridge, MA: MIT Press, 1994), 53.

7 Morten L. Kringelbach et al., "Translational Principles of Deep Brain Stimulation," *Nature Reviews Neuroscience* 8 (August 2007): 623–35.

8   Tipu Aziz quoted in John Harlow, "What a Turn-On: Science Develops Bionic Sex Chip," *Sunday Times* (London), December 21, 2008.

9   Carol L. Baird and Laura Sands, "A Pilot Study of the Effectiveness of Guided Imagery with Progressive Muscle Relaxation to Reduce Chronic Pain and Mobility Difficulties of Osteoarthritis," *Pain Management Nursing* 5, no. 3 (September 2004): 97–104; L. S. Eller, "Guided Imagery Interventions for Symptom Management," *Annual Review of Nursing Research* 17 (1999): 57–84; Alia J. Crum and Ellen Langer, "Mind-Set Matters: Exercise and the Placebo Effect," *Psychological Science* 18, no. 2 (February 2007): 165–71; Erin M. Shackell and Lionel G. Standing, "Mind over Matter: Mental Training Increases Physical Strength," *North American Journal of Psychology* 9, no. 1 (2007): 189–200, www.sportsmindskills.com/images/mind_over_matter_shackell_07.pdf.

10 Mark F. Schwartz and Stephen Southern, "Compulsive Cybersex: The New Tea Room," *Sexual Addiction & Compulsivity* 7, nos. 1–2 (2000): 127–44.

11 Mayo Clinic staff, "Compulsive Sexual Behavior," Mayo Clinic, www.mayoclinic.com/health/compulsive-sexual-behavior/DS00144 (accessed March 2, 2012).

12 Susan Cheever, *Desire: Where Sex Meets Addiction* (New York: Simon & Schuster, 2008).

13 Ibid.

14 Michael Leahy, *Porn University: What College Students Are Really Saying about Sex on Campus* (Northfield, MA: Northfield Publishing, 2009).

Key Three: Express Your Sexuality

Epigraph: Mark Twain in Alex Ayres, ed., *The Wit and Wisdom of Mark Twain* (New York: Harper, 2005), 210.

1   Tara Parker-Pope, "Infidelity Increasing, Especially among Women, Young People," *New York Times*, October 28, 2008.

2   Mark A. Whisman and Douglas K. Snyder, "Sexual Infidelity in a National Survey of American Women: Differences in Prevalence and Correlates as a Function of Method of Assessment," *Journal of Family Psychology* 21, no. 2 (June 2007): 147–54.

3   Helen F. Fisher quoted in Parker-Pope, "Infidelity Increasing."

4   Gary Neuman, "Besides Sex — Other Reasons Men Cheat," Oprah.com, October 2008, www.cnn.com/2008/LIVING/wayoflife/10/03/o.why.men .cheat/index.html (accessed November 2, 2011); Gary Neuman, *The Truth about Cheating: Why Men Stray and What You Can Do to Prevent It* (New York: Wiley, 2008).

5   Cindy M. Meston and David M. Buss, "Why Humans Have Sex," *Archives of Sexual Behavior* 36, no. 4 (August 2007): 477–507.

6   T. R. Insel, "A Neurobiological Basis of Social Attachment," *American Journal of Psychiatry* 154 (June 1997): 726–35; C. S. Carter, "Neuroendocrine Perspectives on Social Attachment and Love," *Psychoneuroendocrinology* 23, no. 8 (November 1998): 779–818.

7   E. M. Brecher, *Love, Sex and Aging: A Consumers Union Report* (Boston: Little, Brown, 1984).

8   Ashley Montagu, *Touching: The Human Significance of the Skin* (New York: Harper & Row, 1971), 99.

9   Ibid., 198.

10 John N. I. Dieter et al., "Stable Preterm Infants Gain More Weight and Sleep Less after Five Days of Massage Therapy," *Journal of Pediatric Psychology* 28, no. 6 (2003): 403–11.

11 Montagu, *Touching*, 206.

12 Ibid., 395.

13 Ibid., xv.

14 Ibid., 181.

15 Debra Bello et al., "An Exploratory Study of Neurohormonal Responses of Healthy Men to Massage," *Journal of Alternative and Complementary Medicine* 14, no. 4 (May 2008): 387–94.

16 Debra Herbenick et al., "Prevalence and Characteristics of Vibrator Use by Women in the United States: Results from a Nationally Representative Study," *Journal of Sexual Medicine* 6, no. 7 (July 2009): 1857–66.

17 Michael Reece et al., "Prevalence and Characteristics of Vibrator Use by Men in the United States," *Journal of Sexual Medicine* 6, no. 7 (July 2009): 1867–74.

18 Michael Reece et al., "Vibrator Use among Heterosexual Men Varies by Partnership Status: Results from a Nationally Representative Study in the United States," *Journal of Sex & Marital Therapy* 36, no. 5 (October 2010): 389–407.

19 Vanessa Schick et al., "Prevalence and Characteristics of Vibrator Use among Women Who Have Sex with Women," *Journal of Sexual Medicine* 8, no. 12 (December 2011): 3306–15.

20 Michael Reece et al., "Characteristics of Vibrator Use by Gay and Bisexually Identified Men in the United States," *Journal of Sexual Medicine* 7, no. 10 (October 2010): 3467–76.

21 Andrea Demirjian, *Kissing: Everything You Ever Wanted to Know about One of Life's Sweetest Pleasures* (self-published, 2006).

22 Michael Penn, *Kissing Christians: Ritual and Community in the Late Ancient Church* (Philadelphia: University of Pennsylvania Press, 2005).

23   Chip Walter, "Affairs of the Lips: Why We Kiss," *Scientific American Mind* (February–March 2008): 27.

24   Peter Kirsch et al., "Oxytocin Modulates Neural Circuitry for Social Cognition and Fear in Humans," *Journal of Neuroscience* 25, no. 49 (December 7, 2005): 11489–93.

25   Paul J. Zak, Robert Kurzban, and William T. Matzner, "Oxytocin Is Associated with Human Trustworthiness," *Hormones and Behavior* 48, no. 5 (December 2005): 522–27.

26   Irwin Goldstein et al., eds., *Women's Sexual Function and Dysfunction: Study, Diagnosis and Treatment* (London: Informa Healthcare, 2005).

27   Marcel D. Waldinger et al., "Ejaculation Disorders: A Multinational Population Survey of Intravaginal Ejaculation Latency Time," *Journal of Sexual Medicine* 2, no. 4 (July 2005): 492–97.

28   Eric W. Corty and Jenay M. Guardiani, "Canadian and American Sex Therapists' Perceptions of Normal and Abnormal Ejaculatory Latencies: How Long Should Intercourse Last?," *Journal of Sexual Medicine* 5, no. 5 (May 2008): 1251–56.

29   "Soy Supplements Cut Sexual Behavior in Rats," *New Scientist*, November 14, 2003, www.newscientist.com.

30   Alison Amsterdam et al., "Persistent Sexual Arousal Syndrome Associated with Increased Soy Intake," *Journal of Sexual Medicine* 2, no. 3 (May 2005): 338–40.

31   Rachel Herz, *The Scent of Desire: Discovering Our Enigmatic Sense of Smell* (New York: HarperPerennial, 2008); Ivanka Savic, Hans Berglund, and Per Lindström, "Brain Response to Putative Pheromones in Homosexual Men," *Proceedings of the National Academy of Sciences* 102, no. 20 (May 17, 2005): 7356–61.

32   Alan Hirsch, "Various Aromas Found to Enhance Male Sexual Response," Smell and Taste Treatment and Research Foundation, www.smellandtaste.org/_/index.cfm?action=research.sexual (accessed March 2, 2012).

33   Mark Moss et al., "Modulation of Cognitive Performance and Mood by Aromas of Peppermint and Ylang-ylang," *International Journal of Neuroscience* 118, no. 1 (January 2008): 59–77.

34   Mark Moss et al., "Aromas of Rosemary and Lavender Essential Oils Differentially Affect Cognition and Mood in Healthy Adults," *International Journal of Neuroscience* 113, no. 1 (January 2003): 15–38.

35   Richard A. Lippa, "The Relation between Sex Drive and Sexual Attraction to Men and Women: A Cross-National Study of Heterosexual, Bisexual, and Homosexual Men and Women," *Archives of Sexual Behavior* 36, no. 2 (April 2007): 209–22.

36 Richard A. Lippa, "Is High Sex Drive Associated with Increased Sexual Attraction to Both Sexes? It Depends on Whether You Are Male or Female," *Psychological Science* 17, no. 1 (January 2006): 46–52.

37 Shaun Brookhouse, "Hypnotherapy and Sexual Dysfunction," www.hypno-nlp.com (accessed November 2, 2011).

38 Daniel L. Araoz and Robert Bleck, *Hypnosex: Sexual Joy through Self-Hypnosis* (New York: Arbor House, 1982).

Key Four: Protect Your Sexuality

Epigraph: Mae West in Michele Brown, ed., *A Collection of Sexy Quotes* (Kansas City, MO: Andrews McMeel, 2006), 3.

1 Michael A. McGeehin, Judith R. Qualters, and Amanda Sue Niskar, "National Environmental Public Health Tracking Program: Bridging the Information Gap," *Environmental Health Perspectives* 112, no. 14 (October 2004): 1409–13; "National Report on Human Exposure to Environmental Chemicals," U.S. Centers for Disease Control and Prevention, www.cdc.gov/exposurereport/ (accessed March 6, 2012).

2 Elizabeth Weise, "Are Our Products Our Enemy?," *USA Today*, August 3, 2005.

3 S. H. Swan et al., "Decrease in Anogenital Distance among Male Infants with Prenatal Phthalate Exposure," *Environmental Health Perspectives* 113, no. 8 (September 2005): 1056–61; Marla Cone, "Study Finds Genital Abnormalities in Boys," *Los Angeles Times*, May 27, 2005.

4 Susan M. Duty et al., "The Relationship between Environmental Exposures to Phthalates and DNA Damage in Human Sperm Using the Neutral Comet Assay," *Environmental Health Perspectives* 111, no. 9 (July 2003): 1164–69.

5 "More Men Seek Breast Reduction," *Sunday Times* (London), July 31, 2005.

6 Randall Fitzgerald, *The Hundred-Year Lie: How to Protect Yourself from the Chemicals That Are Destroying Your Health* (New York: Penguin, 2007), 152–53.

7 Matthew D. Anway and Michael K. Skinner, "Epigenetic Transgenerational Actions of Endocrine Disruptors," *Endocrinology* 147, no. 6 (June 2006): 43–49.

8 Samuel S. Epstein, with Randall Fitzgerald, *Toxic Beauty: How Cosmetics and Personal-Care Products Endanger Your Health…and What You Can Do about It* (Dallas, TX: BenBella Books, 2009), 68–71, 157.

9 Irwin Goldstein et al., eds., *Women's Sexual Function and Dysfunction: Study, Diagnosis and Treatment* (London: Informa Healthcare, 2005).

10 Juha Koskimäki et al., "Regular Intercourse Protects against Erectile Dysfunction: Tampere Aging Male Urologic Study," *American Journal of Medicine* 121, no. 7 (July 2008): 592–96.

11 Roy J. Levin, "The G-Spot — Reality or Illusion?," *Sexual and Relationship Therapy* 18, no.1 (2003): 117–19.

12 Deborah Smith, "Orgasm and the Brain," *Sydney Morning Herald*, April 5, 2007.

13 Terence M. Hines, "The G-Spot: A Modern Gynecologic Myth," *American Journal of Obstetrics & Gynecology* 185, no. 2 (August 2001): 359–62.

14 Karen J. Carlson, Stephanie A. Eisenstat, and Terra Ziporyn, *The New Harvard Guide to Women's Health* (Cambridge, MA: Harvard University Press, 2004).

15 "Poll Reveals Sleep Differences among Ethnic Groups," National Sleep Foundation, March 8, 2010, www.sleepfoundation.org/article/press-release /poll-reveals-sleep-differences-among-ethnic-groups (accessed March 6, 2012).

16 Jenny Hislop, "A Bed of Roses or a Bed of Thorns? Negotiating the Couple Relationship through Sleep," *Sociological Research Online* 12, no. 5 (September 30, 2007).

17 Willard Harley Jr., *Love Busters: Overcoming the Habits That Destroy Romantic Love* (Grand Rapids, MI: Revell, 2007).

18 Michael A. Mangan and Ulf-Dietrich Reips, "Sleep, Sex, and the Web: Surveying the Difficult-to-Reach Clinical Population Suffering from Sexsomnia," *Behavior Research Methods* 39, no. 2 (May 2007): 233–36.

19 N. N. Trajanovic, M. Mangan, and C. M. Shapiro, "Sexual Behaviour in Sleep: An Internet Survey," *Social Psychiatry & Psychiatric Epidemiology* 42, no. 12 (December 2007): 1024–31.

20 Carlos H. Schenck, Isabelle Arnulf, and Mark W. Mahowald, "Sleep and Sex: What Can Go Wrong? A Review of the Literature on Sleep Related Disorders and Abnormal Sexual Behaviors and Experiences," *Sleep* 30, no. 6 (June 2007): 683–702.

21 Carlos H. Schenck quoted in Melinda Wenner, "Have Sex While You Sleep," LiveScience, June 2, 2007, www.livescience.com/health/070602_sleep _oddities.html (accessed November 2, 2011).

22 C. J. Charnetski and F. X. Brennan, "Sexual Frequency and Salivary Immunoglobulin A (IgA)," *Psychological Reports* 94, no. 3, pt. 1 (June 2004): 839–44.

23 Smith, "Orgasm and the Brain."

24 Shari Lieberman quoted in Michael Castleman, "Stop Poisoning Your Sex Life," *Men's Fitness*, March 2003.

Key Five: Nourish Your Sexuality

Epigraph: Elton John in Geoff Tibballs, ed., *The Mammoth Book of Zingers, Quips, and One-Liners* (New York: Caroll & Graf, 2004), 68.

1   D. R. Glenn et al., "Sildenafil Citrate Improves Sperm Motility but Causes a Premature Acrosome Reaction in Vitro," *Fertility and Sterility* 87, no. 5 (May 2007): 1064–70.

2   Ben Hirschler, "Antidepressants May Damage Male Fertility: Study," *Reuters*, September 24, 2008, www.reuters.com/article/2008/09/24/us-antidepressants -sperm-science-idUSTRE48N6L220080924 (accessed March 6, 2012).

3   George L. Redmon, *Sensual for Life: The Natural Way to Maintain Sexual Vitality* (New York: Kensington, 2003), 101; Henry G. Bieler, *Dr. Bieler's Natural Way to Sexual Health* (Boston: Charles Publishing, 1972).

4   Stephen Holt, *The Sexual Revolution* (San Diego: ProMotion Publishing, 1999).

5   Morton Walker, *Sexual Nutrition: How to Nutritionally Improve, Enhance, and Stimulate Your Sexual Appetite* (New York: Avery, 1994).

6   F. Pellestor, A. Girardet, and B. Andreo, "Effect of Long Abstinence Periods on Human Sperm Quality," *International Journal of Fertility & Menopausal Studies* 39, no. 5 (September–October 1994): 278–82.

7   E. Levitas et al., "Relationship between the Duration of Sexual Abstinence and Semen Quality: Analysis of 9,489 Semen Samples," *Fertility & Sterility* 83, no. 6 (June 2005): 1680–86.

8   Emma Wilkinson, "Daily Sex Best for Good Sperm," BBC News, June 30, 2009.

9   L. Bossini et al., "Light Therapy as a Treatment for Sexual Dysfunctions," *Psychotherapy and Psychosomatics* 78, no. 2 (2009): 127–28.

10 L. A. Abramov, "Sexual Life and Sexual Frigidity among Women Developing Acute Myocardial Infarction," *Psychosomatic Medicine* 38, no. 6 (November–December 1976): 418–25.

11 G. G. Gallup Jr., R. L. Burch, and S. M. Platek, "Does Semen Have Antidepressant Qualities?," *Archives of Sexual Behavior* 31, no. 3 (June 2002): 289–93.

12 Roy J. Levin, "Smells and Tastes — Their Putative Influence on Sexual Activity in Humans," *Sexual and Relationship Therapy* 19, no. 4 (November 2004): 451–62.

Key Six: Enhance Your Sexuality

Epigraphs: George Burns in Jack Jacoby, ed., *The Biggest Joke Book Ever* (Victoria, BC: Trafford, 2008), 592; W. C. Fields in Clifton Fadiman, ed., *Bartlett's Book of Anecdotes* (Boston: Little, Brown, 1985), 203.

1   "What Is Tantra?," Tantra.com, www.tantra.com/tantra/what_is_tantra (accessed November 1, 2011).

2   "Watermelon May Have Viagra-Effect," *Science Daily*, June 30, 2008, www .sciencedaily.com/releases/2008/06/080630165707.htm (accessed November 4, 2011).

3   Natasha A. Spencer et al., "Social Chemosignals from Breastfeeding Women
    Increase Sexual Motivation," *Hormones and Behavior* 46, no. 3 (September 2004):
    362–70.

4   Shamshad Ahmad Tajuddin et al., "An Experimental Study of Sexual Function
    Improving Effect of Myristica fragrans Houtt. (Nutmeg)," *BMC Complementary
    and Alternative Medicine* 5, no. 16 (July 20, 2005).

5   Shamshad Ahmad Tajuddin, Abdul Latif, and Iqbal A. Qasmi, "Aphrodisiac
    Activity of 50% Ethanolic Extracts of Myristica fragrans Houtt. (Nutmeg) and
    Syzygium aromaticum (L) Merr. & Perry (Clove) in Male Mice: A Comparative
    Study," *BMC Complementary and Alternative Medicine* 3, no. 6 (October 20, 2003).

6   Sayed Tabrez Ali and Nabeeh I. Rakkah, "Probable Neuro Sexual Mode of Ac-
    tion of Casimiroa edulis Seed Extract versus Sildenafil Citrate (Viagra) on Mating
    Behavior in Normal Male Rats," *Pakistan Journal of Pharmaceutical Sciences* 21,
    no. 1 (January 2008): 1–6.

7   K. Gauthaman, P. G. Adaikan, and R. N. Prasad, "Aphrodisiac Properties of
    Tribulus terrestris Extract (Protodioscin) in Normal and Castrated Rats," *Life
    Sciences* 71, no. 12 (August 2002): 1385–96.

8   J. H. Chiu et al., "Epimedium brevicornum Maxim Extract Relaxes Rabbit
    Corpus Cavernosum through Multitargets on Nitric Oxide / Cyclic Guanosine
    Monophosphate Signaling Pathway," *International Journal of Impotence Research*
    18, no. 4 (July–August 2006): 335–42.

9   "Horny Goat Weed Can Give Viagra a Pretty Hard Time!," *Asian News Interna-
    tional*, September 26, 2008.

10 Mustafa Emre Bakircioglu et al., "Effect of a Chinese Herbal Medicine Mixture
    on a Rat Model of Hypercholesterolemic Erectile Dysfunction," *Journal of Urol-
    ogy* 164, no. 5 (November 2000): 1798–1801.

11 H. K. Choi, D. H. Seong, and K. H. Rha, "Clinical Efficacy of Korean Red Gin-
    seng for Erectile Dysfunction," *International Journal of Impotence Research* 7, no. 3
    (September 1995): 181–86.

12 B. Hong et al., "A Double-Blind Crossover Study Evaluating the Efficacy of Ko-
    rean Red Ginseng in Patients with Erectile Dysfunction: A Preliminary Report,"
    Journal of Urology 168, no. 5 (November 2002): 2070–73.

13 Beverly Whipple quoted in Michael Castleman, "The ArginMax Effect," Salon
    .com, December 5, 2001, www.salon.com/2001/12/05/arginmax/ (accessed
    November 4, 2011).

14 T. Y. Ito et al., "A Double-Blind Placebo-Controlled Study of ArginMax, a
    Nutritional Supplement for Enhancement of Female Sexual Function," *Journal of
    Sex & Marital Therapy* 27 (2001): 541–49.

15 Florence P. Haseltine et al., "Clinical Study of ArginMax, a Nutritional

Supplement for the Enhancement of Female Sexual Function," *Journal of Women's Health* 10, no. 4 (May 2001).

16 Thomas Y. Ito et al., "The Enhancement of Female Sexual Function with Argin-Max, a Nutritional Supplement, among Women Differing in Menopausal Status," *Journal of Sex & Marital Therapy* 32, no. 5 (2006): 369–78.

17 Thomas Y. Ito et al., "The Effects of ArginMax, a Natural Dietary Supplement for Enhancement of Male Sexual Function," *Hawai'i Medical Journal* 57, no. 12 (December 1998): 741.

18 S. Paick and J. H. Lee, "An Experimental Study of the Effect of Ginkgo Biloba Extract on the Human and Rabbit Corpus Cavernosum Tissue," *Journal of Urology* 156, no. 5 (November 1996): 1876–80.

19 Associated Press, "Toad Aphrodisiac Kills Man, NY Issues Warning," MSNBC, May 23, 2008, www.msnbc.msn.com/id/24797206/ns/health-sexual_health/t /toad-aphrodisiac-kills-man-ny-issues-warning/ (accessed November 4, 2011).

20 David J. Weeks, "Sex for the Mature Adult: Health, Self-Esteem and Countering Ageist Stereotypes," *Sexual and Relationship Therapy* 17, no. 3 (August 1, 2002): 231–40.

21 Geoffrey Miller, Joshua M. Tybur, and Brent D. Jordan, "Ovulatory Cycle Effects on Tip Earnings by Lap Dancers: Economic Evidence for Human Estrus?," *Evolution and Human Behavior* 28, no. 6 (November 2007): 375–81.

22 Grace Dorey et al., "Pelvic Floor Exercises for Erectile Dysfunction," *British Journal of Urology International* 96, no. 4 (September 2005): 595–97.

23 Catherine Hood quoted in "Top 10 Natural Ways to Boost Libido," Discovery Health.com, health.howstuffworks.com/sexual-health/sexual-dysfunction /top-10-natural-ways-to-boost-libido.htm (accessed November 4, 2011).

Key Seven: Prolong Your Sexuality

Epigraphs: Charles Bukowski, *More Notes of a Dirty Old Man: The Uncollected Columns* (San Francisco: City Lights Books, 2011); William Shakespeare in John Bartlett, ed., *The Shakespeare Phrase Book* (Boston: Little, Brown, 1881), 947.

1 Merryn Gott and Sharron Hinchliff, "How Important Is Sex in Later Life? The Views of Older People," *Social Science and Medicine* 56, no. 8 (April 2003): 1617–28.

2 John D. DeLamater and Morgan Sill, "Sexual Desire in Later Life," *Journal of Sex Research* 42, no. 2 (May 2005): 138–49.

3 Ronald A. LaTorre and Karen Kear, "Attitudes toward Sex in the Aged," *Archives of Sexual Behavior* 6, no. 3 (1977): 203–13.

4   Mona Wasow and Martin B. Loeb, "Sexuality in Nursing Homes," *Journal of the American Geriatrics Society* 27, no. 2 (February 1979): 73–79.

5   Shirley Damrosch and Janet Cogliano, "Attitudes of Nursing Home Licensed Practical Nurses toward Sexually Active, Older Residents," *Journal of Women & Aging* 6, nos. 1–2 (1994): 123–33.

6   David J. Weeks, "Sex for the Mature Adult: Health, Self-Esteem and Countering Ageist Stereotypes," *Sexual and Relationship Therapy* 17, no. 3 (August 1, 2002): 232.

7   S. Ebrahim et al., "Sexual Intercourse and Risk of Ischaemic Stroke and Coronary Heart Disease: The Caerphilly Study," *Journal of Epidemiology and Community Health* 56, no. 2 (February 2002): 99–102.

8   S. F. Pariser and J. A. Niedermier, "Sex and the Mature Woman," *Journal of Women's Health* 7, no. 7 (September 1998): 849–59.

9   Uwe Hartmann et al., "Low Sexual Desire in Midlife and Older Women: Personality Factors, Psychosocial Development, Present Sexuality," *Menopause* 11, no. 6, pt. 2 (November–December 2004): 726–40.

10 Edward L. Klaiber, *Hormones and the Mind* (New York: HarperCollins, 2002), 33.

11 Susan Rako, *The Hormone of Desire: The Truth about Testosterone, Sexuality and Menopause* (New York: Three Rivers Press, 1999).

12 Mayo Clinic Staff, "Male Menopause: Myth or Reality?," Mayo Clinic, www.mayoclinic.com/health/male-menopause/MC00058 (accessed January 28, 2012).

13 Ernani Luis Rhoden and Abraham Morgentaler, "Risks of Testosterone-Replacement Therapy and Recommendations for Monitoring," *New England Journal of Medicine* 350 (January 29, 2004): 482–92; Marcello Maggio et al., "Relationship between Low Levels of Anabolic Hormones and 6-Year Mortality in Older Men," *Archives of Internal Medicine* 167, no. 20 (November 12, 2007): 2249–54.

14 California Longevity and Vitality Medical Institute, www.drbartnof.com (accessed November 11, 2011).

15 "Intimacy and Sexuality: Toward a Lifespan Perspective," *International Longevity Center — USA, 2006 Workshop Report*, 3.

16 Annie Laura Cotten, "Still Doing It: The Intimate Lives of Women over 65," *Sexual and Relationship Therapy* 20, no. 4 (November 2005): 483–84.

17 George Davey Smith, Stephen Frankel, and John Yarnell, "Sex and Death: Are They Related? Findings from the Caerphilly Cohort Study," *British Medical Journal* 315, no. 7123 (1997): 1641–44.

18 Huang-Kuang Chen et al., "A Prospective Cohort Study on the Effect of Sexual Activity, Libido and Widowhood on Mortality among the Elderly People: 14-Year

Follow-Up of 2,453 Elderly Taiwanese," *International Journal of Epidemiology* 36, no. 5 (June 11, 2007): 1136–42.

19   Weeks, "Sex for the Mature Adult."

20   Mark S. Litwin, "Health Related Quality of Life in Older Men without Prostate Cancer," *Journal of Urology* 161, no. 4 (April 1999): 1180–84.

21   James T. Pacala et al., "Aging Game Improves Medical Students' Attitudes toward Caring for Elders," *Gerontology and Geriatrics Education* 15, no. 4 (1995): 71–81.

22   Ellen J. Langer, *Mindfulness* (Cambridge, MA: DaCapo Press, 1989), 81–113.

23   Ibid., 81–113, 171–95.

24   Bradley Klapper, "Where's the Love? Baby Boomers Unhappy about Sex," *Salt Lake Tribune*, November 22, 2010, www.sltrib.com/sltrib/world/50730649-68 /sex-boomers-percent-women.html.csp (accessed March 2, 2012).

Bibliography

Adcock, Paul. *Jungle King Secrets: A Libido Liberating Lifestyle for Superior Sexual Satisfaction*. Ann Arbor, MI: Loving Healing Press, 2008.

Anand, Margo. *The Art of Sexual Ecstasy*. New York: Tarcher, 1989.

Begley, Sharon. *Train Your Mind, Change Your Brain*. New York: Ballantine, 2007.

Carlson, Karen J., Stephanie A. Eisenstat, and Terra Ziporyn. *The New Harvard Guide to Women's Health*. Cambridge, MA: Harvard University Press, 2004.

Carrellas, Barbara. *Urban Tantra: Sacred Sex for the Twenty-First Century*. Berkeley, CA: Celestial Arts, 2007.

Cheever, Susan. *Desire: Where Sex Meets Addiction*. New York: Simon & Schuster, 2008.

Clement, Brian. *Longevity: Enjoying Long Life without Limits*. Paris: Editions Jouvence, 2006.

Cohen, Ken. *The Essential Qigong Training Course*. Louisville, CO: Sounds True, 2005.

Fischer, Lynn. *The Better Sex Diet*. New York: St. Martin's Paperbacks, 1999.

Flatto, Edwin. *Super Potency: A Doctor's Guide to Better Sex at Any Age*. London: Thorsons, 1991.

Harley, Willard Jr. *Love Busters: Overcoming the Habits That Destroy Romantic Love*. Grand Rapids, MI: Revell, 2007.

Herz, Rachel. *The Scent of Desire: Discovering Our Enigmatic Sense of Smell*. New York: HarperPerennial, 2008.

Hirsch, Alan. *Scentsational Sex*. Rockport, MA: Element Books, 1998.

Klaiber, Edward L. *Hormones and the Mind*. New York: HarperCollins, 2002.

Langer, Ellen J. *Mindfulness*. Cambridge, MA: DaCapo Press, 1989.

Leahy, Michael. *Porn University: What College Students Are Really Saying about Sex on Campus*. Northfield, MA: Northfield Publishing, 2009.

LeVay, Simon. *The Sexual Brain*. Cambridge, MA: MIT Press, 1994.

Mars, Brigitte. *Sex, Love & Health*. North Bergen, NJ: Basic Health Publications, 2002.

Marshall, Fiona. *Natural Aphrodisiacs*. London: Vega, 2003.

McCloskey, Kerry. *The Ultimate Sex Diet*. Englewood, NJ: True Courage Press, 2005.

Mitchell, Deborah. *Nature's Aphrodisiacs: Safe Holistic Approaches to Intensified Sexual Response & Enjoyment*. New York: Dell, 1999.

Montagu, Ashley. *Touching: The Human Significance of the Skin*. New York: Harper & Row, 1986.

Mumford, Jonn. *Ecstasy through Tantra*. St. Paul, MN: Llewellyn, 2005.

Neuman, Gary. *The Truth about Cheating: Why Men Stray and What You Can Do to Prevent It*. New York: Wiley, 2008.

Nickell, Nancy L. *Nature's Aphrodisiacs*. Freedom, CA: Crossing Press, 2001.

Perel, Esther. *Mating in Captivity: Unlocking Erotic Intelligence*. New York: Harper, 2007.

Rako, Susan. *The Hormone of Desire: The Truth about Testosterone, Sexuality and Menopause*. New York: Three Rivers Press, 1999.

Redmon, George L. *Sensual for Life: The Natural Way to Maintain Sexual Health*. New York: Kensington Publishing, 2003.

Schenck, Carlos. *Sleep: A Groundbreaking Guide to the Mysteries, the Problems, and the Solutions*. New York: Avery, 2008.

Shabsigh, Ridwan. *Sensational Sex in 7 Easy Steps*. New York: Rodale, 2007.

Wuh, Hank C. K. *Sexual Fitness*. New York: Perigee, 2002.

Index

About the Authors

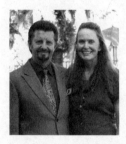 For more than three decades, Brian and Anna Maria Clement have directed The Hippocrates Health Institute in West Palm Beach, Florida, which has been hailed by *Spa Management* magazine as "the number one wellness spa in the world."

More than 300,000 people from fifty countries have spent time at Hippocrates, to strengthen their health using the clinic's holistic model or to heal and recover from illnesses and diseases that mainstream medicine had failed to treat. Among the many dozens of celebrity clients who have lent their names in support of the Hippocrates program are actor Paul Newman, comedian Dick Gregory, and musicians Kenny Loggins and Mick Fleetwood, of Fleetwood Mac.

Drawing upon their training as certified PhD nutritionists, naturopathic medical doctors, and health counselors, and using their natural gifts as dynamic speakers, Brian and Anna Maria Clement lecture on health, nutrition, healing, and longevity before tens of thousands of people internationally each year. Brian has made appearances before the United Nations in Geneva and is a founding director of the Coalition of Holistic Health, which includes numerous national and international health organizations. Their website is www.hippocratesinstitute.org.

They share a longtime loving marriage, are the parents of four children, and have, so far, two grandchildren.

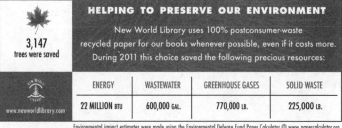

HELPING TO PRESERVE OUR ENVIRONMENT

New World Library uses 100% postconsumer-waste recycled paper for our books whenever possible, even if it costs more. During 2011 this choice saved the following precious resources:

3,147
trees were saved

www.newworldlibrary.com

	ENERGY	WASTEWATER	GREENHOUSE GASES	SOLID WASTE
	22 MILLION BTU	600,000 GAL.	770,000 LB.	225,000 LB.

Environmental impact estimates were made using the Environmental Defense Fund Paper Calculator @ www.papercalculator.org.